Seriously! Garlic?

The Covid Trials of a Naturopathic Physician

By Rick Marschall

Health/Medical Disclaimer

The author and publisher are providing this book and its contents on an "as is" basis. They make no representations or warranties of any kind with respect to this book or its contents. The author and publisher disclaim all such representations and warranties, including for example warranties of merchantability and healthcare for a particular purpose. In addition, the author and publisher do not represent or warrant that the information accessible via this book is accurate, complete or current.

The statements made about products and services have not been evaluated by the US Food and Drug Administration. They are not intended to diagnose, treat, cure, or prevent any condition or disease. Please consult with your own physician or healthcare specialist regarding the suggestions and recommendations made in this book.

Except as specifically stated in this book, neither the author nor publisher, nor any authors, contributors, nor other representatives will be liable for damages arising out of or in connection with the use of this book. This is a comprehensive limitation of liability that applies to all damages of any kind, including (without limitation) compensatory; direct, indirect or consequential damages; loss of data, income or profit; loss of or damage to property and claims of third parties.

Understand that this book is not intended as a substitute for consultation with a licensed healthcare practitioner, such as your physician. Before you begin any healthcare program, or change your lifestyle in any way, you will consult your physician or another licensed healthcare practitioner to ensure that you are in good health and that the examples contained in this book will not harm you.

This book provides content related to physical and/or mental health issues. As such, use of this book implies your acceptance of this disclaimer.

Acknowledgements

I want to thank my dear wife, Rose, who has been there all along cheering me on and taking any and every opportunity to help me counter the constitutionally vapid and greedy Big Pharma driven federal officials who have taken part in this travesty of justice. I am also very lucky to have four wonderful children, who all shared with me individually how unjust and wrong they believe this action was.

I also want to thank the people who traveled to the Tacoma, Washington, Federal Courthouse to observe the trials or give supportive testimony on my behalf:

- Elliot Cohen, a staunch proponent of medical freedom, who flew all the way from Arizona for a trial and who presented me with new research on garlic and Covid
- Ken Morris, my old friend and former band mate from Port Angeles who has always been a loyal supporter
- David and Marianne Boone from Brinnon, who supported me spiritually and in many other ways
- Mark Lamden ND, my oldest, close friend and colleague
- Eric Yarnell N.D. professor of Botanical Medicine at Bastyr University who presented the most thorough explanation of

the benefits of garlic to infectious disease to the jury I could have ever hoped for

I want to thank people who supported me in special ways:

- Gerald Baude, who spent considerable time editing my book and advising me on ways to improve its organization and content, Gerald has been instrumental in making this book get out to the public. His work with the Health Freedom Information group, Informed Consent Washington, and his oversight of the Washington Department of Health has established him as a tireless servant of the health changes we all in America need to see happen.
- Jodi Wilke, who worked so hard to start the GiveSendGo donations account that helped Rose and me survive the time apart financially. She was an angel sent from

above that supported the two of us when we needed it most.
- Laura Roberts, a very dear supportive friend who gave me key insights into how to present this book in an open-minded light to draw even hard core skeptics into understanding these issues.
- Scott Tips, the president of the National Health Federation; Rose contacted him after my conviction to see whether he was interested in publishing my story in the NHF quarterly journal Health Freedom News. Scott patiently waited for me to send him the bullet points of this saga, which I sent him while in the halfway house. His story came out in the winter edition of early 2023. Scott did a great write-up. He is a cool person, a tireless protector of health freedom and a real pro.
- Many thanks go to my friends at the Health Freedom Information Group on the North Olympic Peninsula. These men and women

have stood by me and supported me on a weekly basis as I have gone through this ordeal. These 20-30 people of the North Olympic Peninsula in Washington State are like the three percent of American colonists who actually did something when the British government overstepped their rule and tried to make financial and oppressed slaves of the people living in the thirteen colonies. You 'three-percenters" rock!

I also want to thank people all over the United States who supported me with letters I received while I was in prison and through communications presented to me before going in while I was in the halfway house: my lifelong partner Rose Marschall, my dear siblings Steve Marschall, Teresa Weatherly and Tom Marschall, my nephew Stephen Marschall, my children Barry, Paul, Jon Marschall, and Claire Ongna, the caring Dubbers from Alaska, my dear colleagues Karen Hunter and Mark Lamden, the long time supportive Grahams from Florida, and from my home town true believers, Paris Humble and Brian Booren. In the prison camp, we received mail only two times a week. From the faces and the comments of other inmates, I could see that I was the luckiest man there because when I showed up to the mail drop area I usually had the largest pile.

I also want to give special thanks to my daughter Claire and my sons Paul, Jon and Barry who supported me with compassionate concern as this fiasco unfolded and/or in attendance at my trials.

These family members, friends, patients and colleagues have always known the truth about what has happened. Their support and loyalty has meant more to me than they will ever know.

Preface

This book has several different purposes:

- To tell the story of how I was charged, indicted, put on trial twice, convicted, sentenced and incarcerated for early treatment of Covid-19.
- To share the science of how the Covid-19 virus pandemic came to be
- To share the facts regarding the creation and safety of the Covid-19 "vaccine."
- To share how both vaccinated and unvaccinated people can protect them in this brave new post pandemic world.

Introduction

I'm seventy two years old now. I have thirty-two years of family practice naturopathic medicine behind me treating people with plant-based medicine, nutriceuticals, homeopathics, hydrotherapy, proper diet and exercise. I also have 6 years of health coaching practice since my license was retired by the FDA driven tag team of the Naturopathic Board and the Washington Board of Health as you will learn about later.

I was a free man until July of 2022 when I surrendered to a Federal Prison Camp in Oregon. My only alternative to that would have been to go on the run from the federal government or move to a more compassionate country like Norway or England. I chose to stay and continue the fight for the future health of my American patients and for the health freedom of all other Americans. After serving half of my eight-month sentence in a federal prison, I continued my incarceration at a different federal facility known as a half-way house in Tacoma, Washington to finish the eight months, with the ability to go home two days each week. All this incarceration foolishness by the Federal judge and the FDA in the hopes that I would be rehabilitated from the crime I was convicted of you shall soon understand.

I began this book in early November 2022 when I was sitting in the halfway house in Tacoma, Washington, five days a week with pretty much nothing to do so but exercise. I decided to write the story of Garlic Rick, the handle given to me by prison camp inmates. You might be wondering, what terrible crime a high-powered federal prosecutor charged this physician of thirty four years with to warrant his eventual eight-month incarceration in the federal prison system? Are you a little curious as to why a federal judge gave him an eight-month sentence? Ah! It is a story rather difficult to imagine and somewhat unique in the annals of the FDA and the United States Department of Justice. In these pages you will learn about how about two million taxpayer dollars were misspent to protect you from this harmless physician who helped people survive and thrive in the early days of Covid-19. This is my story.

Chapter 1

The Background for the Crime

In 2020, people started coming down with the usual and unusual flu. By March it was obvious to physicians all over the world that this flu was much more difficult to treat…in fact, there **was** no effective treatment and hospital treatment from the beginning often made the victims of this disease more debilitated. What is worse, more people died from this new flu than had ever died in a typical year from the usual flu.

As we all know, treatment for the regular flu is water, rest and vitamin C, which works more often than not and generally keeps flu victims from going to the hospital. However, treatment for this unusual flu was so ineffective that by the end of 2020 over 375,000 Americans had died during this one flu season, some from the usual flu but most from a flu named Covid-19. They named it Covid-19 because the first cases appeared in the Wuhan district of China at the beginning of the flu season in late 2019 and this virus resembled the natural wild Coronavirus found in dogs, rabbits, bats, pangolins and other animals.

As early as January of 2020, this Covid-19 flu went on a plane trip. It spread from China to northern Italy, New York City, Chicago, Los Angeles, Washington state, Texas and Arizona. Washington State, my niche of the woods, recorded the very first deaths of two people living in a long-term care facility in Kirkland Washington. In a typical flu season in the United States, you will find that the number of people who die is generally between forty and sixty thousand. Usually these flu deaths occur in the immune-compromised elderly, overmedicated patients of all ages, people on recreational drugs and rarely very young children whose immune systems are not fully developed or compromised for some other reason.

This unusual flu caused most of its deaths only in the elderly, especially seniors with heart disease, diabetes, cancer, and autoimmune diseases. Young adults, middle-aged adults and children were almost never victims of Covid-19.

What was different about the Covid-19 flu? This new flu did not just cause inflammation in the lungs and nasal passages; it caused blood clots, loss of smell and taste, damage to the hemoglobin molecule in the red blood cell, damage to the heart muscle cells, and major lung tissue inflammation. It did not respond well to anti-inflammatory drugs, antibiotics, or artificial ventilation.

It was also clear to any physician or scientist paying attention at the onset of 2020 that the wild corona virus did not magically cross over from bats or pangolins in 2019 after living in animals who in turn have lived amongst humans for the last several thousand years rarely ever crossing over to cause human disease. Remember, the usual flu on the average killed only a fraction of those killed by Covid-19. If you simply subtract the worst flu year death toll (60,000) in the United States from the 375,000 Covid deaths by the end of 2020, the extra flu deaths come to 315,000 deaths over and above the usual flu deaths in the United States. The usual flu for the most part caused deaths only during the harshest time of the year when weather was cold and indoor air dry. This new virus kept on killing Americans throughout 2020 and 2021, even when the weather was warmer.

Then there is the PCR test fraud. In the spring of 2020, testing became available for Covid-19. The testing was so inaccurate that by the summer of 2021 test kits were being recalled by the FDA for false positives, tests saying you had it when you did not. As an example, one of my sons living in the Seattle area went to a major hospital to have elective elbow surgery in the summer of 2020. He walked into the hospital with zero Covid symptoms but tested positive for Covid-19. Nevertheless, they rescheduled him for surgery two weeks later, causing him an extended period of loss of range of motion and making it harder for him to do his job. The same day he was tested positive for Covid at the hospital, his twin sister a nurse, was visiting from California. She had some Covid-19 test kits with her and tested him within a day. Both of these tests results showed he did NOT have Covid-19. He subsequently drove to two other hospitals to get tested in the next 24 hours only to continue finding he was negative for Covid. This is a story so common that if you have not heard of it yet you are living in a van down by the river.

Then there is the Covid-19 death certificate fraud. Scott Tips, president of the Natural Health Federation weighs in on this issue: "In February

2020, the World Health Organization (WHO) – never known for its accuracy or consistency – declared a "Pandemic" for the corona virus and claimed that the mortality rate for the novel (new) corona virus disease, now designated as "COVID-19" was 3.4 percent, while that for the seasonal flu was 0.1 percent. Of course, the news media ran with those numbers and splashed scary headlines across the world stating how much more deadly this new virus was than the seasonal flu. The problem with the W.H.O.'s statement was that it applied two different formulas for the two viruses. For the COVID-19 disease, for example, W.H.O simply didn't count any of the mild cases of COVID-19 that resolved by themselves; yet, it did with the seasonal flu. If the W.H.O were to apply the same formula to seasonal flu cases as it did with COVID-19 cases, then the seasonal flu is revealed more truthfully as being twice as deadly as the COVID-19 virus. In fact, the Center for Disease Control and Prevention (CDC) itself has stated that for the 2019-2020 flu seasons, 24-62,000 Americans have died of the seasonal flu, while it has claimed that 53,922 Americans have died of COVID-19 flu as of April 26, 2020." [1]

And for all of this, our Federal, State and local governments are willing to trash the American economy and destroy domestic and international financial markets, most of which are based on the US dollar? In addition, why now? We must ask ourselves these questions because this drastic approach was not adopted during earlier epidemics with far more deadly viruses. So, why now?

Later on in Scot's excellent analysis of this issue he asks his readers to: "follow the money." "In its COVID-19 Alert No. 2 (March 24, 2020), the CDC issued a directive to medical personnel that actually states, "COVID-19 should be reported on the death certificate for all decedents where the disease

---

[1] Tips, Scott. "Never Has So Little Done So Much Harm to So Many." *Health Freedom News*, vol. 38, no. No. 1, 2020, p. 7.

caused or is **assumed to have caused or contributed to death.**"²

It is easy to see that official death figures from COVID-19 are exaggerated and that doctors may assign the virus as a cause of death even without having tested the patient! Moreover, in the United States, there is a financial incentive for hospitals to declare a patient "COVID-19 positive", since the government will reimburse the hospital much more for such patients. For example, at the end of a difficult case of the common flu, a bill of $10-13,000 would accrue. If the patient was diagnosed with Covid-199 the bill could easily accrue to $35-40,000, three times more.

Scott goes on to report: "Then, on March 26th, an article appeared in the New England Journal of Medicine, co-authored by the now-celebrity-status Covid mogul, Dr. Anthony Fauci, which says in a

---

² Tips, Scott. "Never Has So Little Done So Much Harm to So Many." *Health Freedom News*, vol. 38, no. No. 1, 2020, p. 8.

pertinent part, "If one assumes that the number of asymptomatic or minimally symptomatic cases is several times as high as the number of reported cases, the case fatality rate may be considerably less than 1 percent".[3]

This suggests that the overall clinical consequences of Covid-19 may ultimately be more akin to those of a severe seasonal influenza, (which has a case fatality rate of approximately 0.1 percent) (*Health Freedom News / Spring 2020*) or a pandemic influenza (similar to those in 1957 and 1968) rather than a disease similar to SARS or MERS, which had case fatality rates of 9 to 10 percent and 36 percent, respectively.[4]

---

[3] Tips, Scott. "Never Has So Little Done So Much Harm to So Many." *Health Freedom News*, vol. 38, no. No. 1, 2020, p. 8.

[4] https://www.nejm.org/doi/full/10.1056/nejme2002387

Currently CDC sources would have you believe that 1,188,991 Americans have died from Covid-19 since April of 2020 through April of 2024. We will never know how many people in the United States have actually died of Covid-19 rather than the many other chronic diseases they were already suffering from that the Coronavirus made worse. This is because hospital administrators and staff doctors were encouraged to put Covid-19 as the cause of death if the patients tested positive, if they ended up dying while in the hospital. This includes cases where the patient had no symptoms of Covid-19 at all when they were admitted and throughout their stay. We can also easily hypothesize that during 2020 many of the deaths attributed to Covid-19 actually occurred from lack of early treatment of someone who actually **had** the symptoms later recognized as specific to Covid-19. Often these patients, too frightened by the stories of suffering and death they heard that patients went through that went to the hospital often remained home allowing the disease process to progress to a point where it became difficult to treat, especially since the CDC had no effective treatment to offer in the hospitals. One must understand that many primary care doctors, family physicians and general practitioners were avoiding even treating these patients from their clinics because they were scared to do so or because they simply didn't know what to do.

Then, as 2020 April progressed, the CDC, FDA, and the State Boards of Health were arduously intimidating physicians from using any off-label treatments. This was the most egregious oppression I have ever known in my medical years, to see so many Americans dying of ineffectual hospital treatments using Vancomycin, Dexamethasone and ventilators that consistently failed with patients who had Covid-19. All the time America saw a few outpatient physicians like myself, standing up to this mindless and cruel forbidding of natural and safe plant based early treatments and then by June, off-label pharmaceuticals treatments that were saving lives all throughout 2020 and beyond.

Considering the oppressive nature of the FDA, Big Pharma and Big Jurisprudence, you can bet we will hear in from Big Press of how many people have died from taking garlic and larch starch, or hydroxychloroquin and Ivermectin, if there ever is one. I personally started using my garlic and larch starch immediately after symptoms started to appear in February of 2020. To this day in May of 2024, no one has ever died from Covid-19 on my watch.

Unfortunately, the talking heads, the so called experts of Covid-19, Anthony Fauci and Deborah Birx, members of the media especially CNN, the government mouthpiece called the Center for Disease Control (CDC) and its counterparts in the European Health agencies, the World Health Organization (W.H.O) from the beginning, seemed to have chosen to ignore the scientific facts as they gradually presented themselves.[5] Instead, they began by telling us this corona virus was a "novel"

---

[5] https://www.brown-watch.com/brownwatch-news/2021/8/4/sdsds

virus. Novel means it was new to humans. They convinced many people that a bat virus containing a "mutated" corona virus suddenly crossed over to humans in the Wuhan district of China and simply traveled around the world as Chinese people traveled abroad, killing people in foreign countries by spreading it from one culture to another. This certainly appeared to be a lie right from the start to virtually any scientist or physician paying attention. Not an "Oops, we didn't get it right, and we're sorry" kind of mistake but apparently a lie calculated to cover up a fact.[6]

When you first heard these statements about the probable bat/pangolin virus crossover by certain medical authorities like Fauci, Birx, the WHO and others, what did your gut tell you? Did the epidemic in Wuhan district convince you an animal virus appeared "out of thin air," and started killing elderly Chinese and later your parents and

---

[6] https://www.brown-watch.com/brownwatch-news/2021/8/4/sdsds

grandparents? Did Fauci provide ANY evidence that a bat virus was the cause? No, it's clear now that Fauci did not show evidence, and it's clear now he only presented the bat/pangolin source as a diversion. He knew most people would not check into the history of the natural corona virus or **his history of bioengineering**. He sold the world a story without providing any facts and once people started getting sick, very sick, he figured he had everyone's attention appearing as the wise old scientist and towards the end of 2020 encouraged people to wait for an up and coming vaccine that would fix everything.[7]

As the 2020 pandemic unfolded, like me, you would have preferred to be presented with scientific facts from our health authorities about the origin of the virus and the effective outpatient treatments available as evidence came in, regardless of who and what was actually responsible. Instead, the

---

[7] https://www.brown-watch.com/brownwatch-news/2021/8/4/sdsds

truth about the cause of the pandemic was kept a secret.

As you will shortly see, the truth is plain to see in the written evidence collected by the Federal government that the director of the government's own infectious disease agency, Anthony Fauci, bioengineered a virus over a twenty year period. This virus he knows was capable of killing millions of people around the world and setting the stage for Big Pharma to start injecting people with a new technology.[8] Hold on, I know what you're thinking. Why in God's name would the highest infectious disease authority in the greatest and most powerful nation in the world want the cause the spread of a deadly virus and even more deadly vaccine? It's hard to even comprehend the possibility right? When this notion first entered my brain after watching a interview by an attorney of David Malone M.D. who proved beyond a shadow of

---

[8] https://www.brown-watch.com/brownwatch-news/2021/8/4/sdsds

doubt that Fauci was directly responsible for creating the deadly Covid-19 bioengineered virus, I still didn't want to believe it. But my friends, read on and if you can find a hole in this narrative, please email me as I'm willing to learn.

Always keep in mind, while you, your family, friends and coworkers were home sick or dying in hospitals all across America, physicians who were willing to treat you **before** you needed the Intensive Care Unit (ICU) were threatened with the loss of their license. To make this work your local pharmacist was ordered **not** to fill the prescriptions of physicians. This government repression of brave physicians willing to risk their professional reputations, financial livelihoods, hospital contracts, medical licenses and personal freedoms should always be in the back of your mind when you are attempting to decide at any future point in your life if you actually trust your government to have your best interests in mind.

Later, in January 2021 when the government gave emergency use to the first vaccine, I am sure all Americans wanted to understand the evidence for this vaccine's safety and effectiveness. If all these things were your preference, take the red pill and I will provide you with the evidence for what the government has done. If not take the blue pill, lean back on your lazy boy, turn the television to the corporate media channels and continue to accept the story you have been told by officials who swear to have your best interest at heart. Continue to go to the government websites that presented the statistics in 2020 about the unusual Covi-19 flu while they never once mentioned the statistics about the usual flu, as if the regular influenza virus simply disappeared off the face of the earth. Continue to get boosters and believe they will stop Covid-19, even after you or someone you know comes down with the symptoms of Covid-19 within days, weeks or months after being vaccinated. Continue to wear masks while viral particles slip right past them and enter your lungs. Continue to do whatever your government tells you to do for the rest of your life.

Looking past the lies means you have to follow the research, think logically, and use critical thinking skills and wake up to the truth. It is not for everyone and physicians like myself have as much compassion for the fearful mRNA vaccine takers as we do for the brave Americans who refused the vaccine, whether they did it in January 2021 or finally stopped accepting boosters anytime thereafter.

Did you notice that by November 2022, the government and corporate -sponsored CNN, ABC and other "yes sir!" types began changing their tune? After the 2020-2021 influenza free-years, they began telling people that during the winter of 2021, the usual flu vaccine would become available again, and you should take it because miraculously, government experts had determined that it was no longer hibernating, it's back!

As I watched all this unfold in the first 2 months of 2020, I realized something was really wrong for the first time in the history of American medicine. Of course I didn't have all the facts because it hadn't played out quite yet but this new pandemic virus didn't feel like any of the previous incarnation of a coronavirus like SARS or MERS. Something was up! I knew I had to be ready to treat people regardless of how the government was going to play this out so I got ready.

Chapter 2

My Early Treatment of Covid-19

Covid-19 came to America very quickly, all across the states as I have mentioned above. No one had an adequate treatment for the seriously ill. Even in the hospital, many died, not learning their lessons from the SARS outbreak of 2009 or the MERS outbreak of 2014 when it became clear that a coronavirus should **not** be treated with a ventilator. By the time it was realized that unlike SARS and MERS, this corona virus was going to be very lethal in February of 2020, there was as yet no approved treatment for a coronavirus. In other words, after eleven years, modern medical science had no effective treatment for all versions of the corona virus SARS, MERS and now Covid.

I have a four year naturopathic medical degree from Bastyr University in the Seattle area. I received an extra 1,000 hours of training compared to a medical doctor because I had two full years of nutrition as well as being required to have as much training in pharmaceuticals and everything else that is taught in any conventional medical school. I did an internship and a two year residency in family practice. I was in private practice for thirty-two years. I have never been sued nor had a malpractice case. All physicians receive complaints during some decades of practice. All five complaints I received during those thirty-two years submitted to the Washington Department of Health were deemed unsubstantiated and closed. If you call the Washington State Department of Health and ask them if I have ever harmed anyone in my entire career they will tell you no like they told me. My license was revoked in 2018 only because after sending patients out of state their natural medicines against the FDA's statues. I did this knowingly continuing to support patients in other states with their healthcare, sending them whatever natural treatments they required and the FDA didn't like that. It didn't matter to me that their statutes were created to hinder physicians from caring for their patients who had moved to other states in our union. It didn't matter to me that the FDA, an agency willing to ignore the constitution if it helped them redirect the attention of the American people away from alternative medicine at the behest of Big Pharma and to protect the AMA's hold over all medical care.

As an example of this, I found out early on that the FDA had no problem with MDs practicing "Telemedicine," but they treated alternative physicians like me as a sort of "nuisance" physician, the uncle you wished you had not invited to the party. The FDA had no jurisdiction in Washington State to take away my license. They did have the powerful Federal government's clout to influence the Washington Department of Health to convince them to de-license me after 32 years of harmless, faithful, successful service to thousands of Americans. Again, explain to me how I've made a false statement because I'm willing to learn. Luckily, the Washington Department of Health said to me afterwards in no uncertain terms that I could practice as a health coach without any state supervision of any kind. Therefore, since I had no intention of moving to any of several states who were offering me a license I have continued to practice legally as Rick Marschall ND, health coach. I thought carefully about the opportunity of moving to another state like Montana, Oregon. I decided against it for two reasons, the main one being and didn't want to move away from where my children resided and the other...I just wasn't going to let these arrogant fools dictate my options. The cool thing was, I hadn't prescribed anything at all in about 6 years. I could continue helping people overcome diseases and conditions by coaching them on the use of proper vegetarian diet, plant based substances and other non-drug or surgical interventions when possible. And I've been doing this successfully as a health coach for the last six years without any obstruction by the DOH. As the office manager at the State of Washington Department of Health (DOH) had made it clear, I was no longer under the jurisdiction of the DOH and as long as I didn't harm anyone or prescribe anything they had no cause to bother me.

It's funny but, losing the license gave way to incremental feelings of relief. Relief from the anxiety of supervisorial pressure by a spineless agency of my own state government led to a sense of relaxation that continues today.

In late February of 2020, I found my dear wife Rose on the second day of her illness still lying on the couch, quite sick from what appeared to be a very bad flu. To be fair to Rose I do not remember seeing her being sick from more than a short-lived cold for many years. She said she had been taking the special garlic preparation I use, Stabilized Allicin, a very broad spectrum and potent antimicrobial that has worked well for the usual viral flu. She took this along with IAG, a larch tree starch powder immune booster, both of which I have been using for over thirty years. I asked her how much she was taking and she said two capsules of the garlic and a teaspoon of the larch powder. I replied that she had not been ill in so long that apparently she had forgot the standard dose. I brought her seven capsules of Stabilized Allicin 7 mg. and a tablespoon of IAG powder in some warm water. By that evening, she was feeling much better and in the morning, she was back to normal.

Rose to this day believes she had Covid-19. It certainly is a possibility. Shortly thereafter, she posted her experience to Facebook. If you have experience with Facebook, sometimes you might allow a person who acts like a friend to become part of your 'friend' group. We found out later from our attorneys the names of two people in our community that had complained to the Washington State Department of Health from her post that Rose and I were promoting early treatment of Covid-19 with this special preparation of garlic and larch starch!

Eventually her success with these two natural treatments went from the Washington Department of Health to the FDA prosecutor looking to save the public from "Covid-19 misinformation," that is, early treatments for Covid-19. How arrogant can one agency be? The government admitted there was no approved or known effective treatment for Covid-19 from the very beginning of 2020. People were dying in large numbers in hospitals all over the United States. So why did the federal government get their panties in a twist when the citizens these government officials have the privilege of serving, decided to seek to treat this deadly virus with anything 'generally recognized as safe' (GRAS) at all?

It is of paramount importance readers that you remember that at this point there was no effective treatment for Covid-19. There was no harm in taking a garlic or larch tree preparation when the consequences of doing nothing or going to the hospital and dying from vancomycin, prednisone and a ventilator were much worse. This is straightforward common sense, right?

The US Constitution, our contract with the federal government, was built on common sense, common law going back to the Magna Carta. According to our constitution, there is no crime if there is no harm done. Let that sink in. Every American has the constitutional right to use a GRAS product for any condition or speak of the use of any GRAS product through the First Amendment freedom of speech. Every American has the right to ship to any other American living in any other state these natural medicines due to the Commerce clause written in the body of the Constitution itself. The statutes the FDA uses to harm innocent American citizens on the other hand are contrived by this agency to overrule the Constitution of the United States of America. Our US Constitution has been corrupted by multiple federal agencies beginning with the 1860s. Almost every senior American knows this when they watched the FDA raid alternative doctor Jonathan Wright MD's office in 1992 with flak jackets, guns drawn and using a ram to smash through his front door. They were in search of a harmless amino acid tryptophan that is to this day successfully used in the treatment of schizophrenia. I remember when I was premed living in Northern California watching James Privitera MD in handcuffs and shackles led away from his home for safely and effectively using pancreatic enzymes and an apricot kernel extract in the treatment of cancers that chemotherapy had failed.

Do nothing and die or take a natural product. Avoid ineffective toxic drugs and the ventilator and possibly survive. Many people have been taking natural products during Covid-19 to avoid the danger of dying in the local hospitals. The FDA certainly didn't go after them. They have a constitutional right to do so as I have substantiated above. This common law common sense fact was reiterated by former president Donald Trump during the pandemic. He reminded Americans of their (constitutional) 'Right to Try' any treatment that was generally recommended as safe (GRAS) and possibly effective, if they experienced the symptoms of Covid-19. President Trump treated himself with hydroxychloroquine and other GRAS remedies when he experienced Covid symptoms in 2020.

How does Stabilized Allicin work against Covid-19? First, Stabilized Allicin, an extract of garlic, is a unique product that originally came from Europe. Health researchers have studied garlic extracts for over 100 years. When you eat garlic, you chew two compartments of the garlic plant. One compartment contains alliin; the other compartment contains an enzyme that converts the alliin into allicin. Alliin helps reduce cholesterol and lower blood pressure. Allicin has potent antimicrobial properties. It has shown effectiveness against many different viruses, bacteria, parasites including worms, yeast including Candida, and other microbes. There is strong clinical and double-blind placebo evidence for this natural medicine.

Allicin can also repair the hemoglobin molecule. As the pandemic continued, Covid-19 showed us its ability to damage the person's oxygen carrying red blood cells made of hemoglobin. This is why allicin has been so effective against Covid-19. Remdesvir may destroy some of the Covid-19 viruses but at the expense of the kidney, and it does not repair the critical oxygen carrying hemoglobin. Furthermore there is evidence that Remdesivir like other antiviral drugs appears to cause damage to the oxygen carrying red blood cell system by an unknown mechanism.[9]

Stabilized Allicin is not like the garlic powder you buy in the grocery store. It is not like garlic oil. This product is prepared from taking many cloves of garlic and washing them in such a way as to liberate the allicin extract. When you eat raw garlic much of the aliin isn't converted to allicin because the enzyme that converts it is destroyed by stomach acid. The process for concentrating the allicin took years to develop. The dose of Stabilized Allicin for a typical infection at seven milligrams is seven

---

[9]https://www.ncbi.nlm.nih.gov/pmc/articles/PMC9263052/#:~:text=Moreover%2C%20Nabil%20et%20al.',COVID%2D19%20%5B67%5D.

capsules for a 150-220 pound adult every twelve hours until better. Granted, that is many pills to take but plant medicines are made from whole foods and it often takes more substance to treat an illness than the small amount of chemical required from a tiny synthetic drug pill.

How does IAG powder work? IAG stands for inulo-arabino-galactan. It's a long fancy name for the starch living under the Larch tree bark. Larch trees grow all over the United States and there are many in the Cascade Mountains here in my state of Washington. The American Indians living in the mountains east of Seattle used the larch tree for medicine before white people ever came here. They would skin some bark from a larch tree, wash the starch from it with water and drink the concoction. American physicians going back to the origins of this country conducted empirical studies on the effectiveness of larch starch on infections. An empirical study is a kind of therapeutic trial. There is no control group, they would simply give a preparation of larch starch to a group of infected subjects and see if they improved. There are many more recent scientific studies published on Pub Med on the ability of Larch tree IAG to increase killer T-cells that attack and destroy viruses. Therefore, while IAG does not have direct antiviral activity, it does boost the persons own immune systems specific cells that destroy viruses. IAG is also a decongestant, something that helps remove products of inflammation in the lungs and upper respiratory tract.

Well, the word got out. Friends, family, and former patients started taking Stabilized Allicin and IAG powder when they came down with Covid-19 symptoms. They got better, some within twenty-four hours, others took longer depending on their general state of immune health at the time they showed the first symptoms. Furthermore, not one of my people died no matter how severe their symptoms were. None of them went to the hospital either. It was also logical to them that they had done a smart thing because by doing so they never had to consider even entering the emergency room. They thank God and nature every day that this treatment came into their life because a look at the success of Covid-19 hospitalizations shows that they are rather lucky to be alive.

If what I was doing during the early days of Covid-19 was dangerous, then the federal prosecutor should have put me in some detention center while I was awaiting trial. He did not. For almost two full years, I was allowed to continue to practice as a health coach, making Stabilized Allicin and IAG powder available to hundreds of people. That's also not counting the even larger group of people who were saved from this disease, suffering and death when they shared this knowledge with friends, family or patients.

People were suffering from what appeared to the patient to be Covid-19. Often their condition was declared by a medical official as Covid-19 based on the questionable PCR test. If you remember, in

2020 and later during the pandemic, the medical authorities from the CDC and FDA decided to recall the PCR test kits due to mixed results. For example, some people tested positive but have no symptoms while in other cases people had symptoms but a negative test result. But cases I was involved with, where the victim could not taste or smell, was to me the most reliable test for Covid-19. Since the regular flu was still around and the PCR test was unreliable, losing your taste or smell was and is the most reliable symptom for a person to confirm a person has Covid-19.

To reiterate the outcomes, no one ever died and most got better relatively quickly from this natural treatment. Usually with only one to four recommended doses. Later on two controlled studies showing the positive effects of Allicin specifically against Covid-19 were published.[10] [11]

10

https://www.frontiersin.org/articles/10.3389/fmicb.2021.746795/full

Unbeknownst to most Americans at the time, the Federal Trade Commission (FTC) had just created a statute designed to thwart physicians willing to provide early treatment for Covid-19, even though there was no targeted, effective treatment offered for this "new" virus. The first physician to receive a warning letter by the FTC was Dr. Eric Nepute from the St. Louis, Missouri, area. He received the warning a week before I was notified by the Federal Prosecutor as you will see. Was I sent such a letter? No. Both Dr. Nepute and I were doing the same thing, offering alternative treatment for Covid-19. Dr. Nepute received a warning letter and I was charged with a felony.[12]

On May 27, 2020, I got an email from the federal prosecutor's office charging me with "misbranding

---

11
https://www.ncbi.nlm.nih.gov/pmc/articles/PMC8274222/

12 https://www.webmd.com/lung/news/20210422/first-person-charged-under-covid-false-claims-law

of a drug in interstate commerce." Crazy, huh? Misbranding a nutritional garlic supplement as a drug? How do you do that with garlic, a non-toxic, nutritional supplement? A year later the Government (FDA) approves Remdesvir, a toxic, lethal drug. Go figure. Worse than that, it seemed like the prosecutor was simply an arm of Big Pharma, the Deep State and Fauci who was working up his mojo to offer the toxic drug Remdesvir in January of 2021?

It sure seemed like our federal government decided they had to stop the possible emergence of safe and natural early treatments of Covid-19 during 2020, an entire year before hospitals around the country had even one anti-viral medicine approved or even "tested" on sick or dying Covid-19 patients. People do not die after taking garlic and larch tree starch. They certainly died in the hospitals in 2020 from their treatments using Dexamethasone as the anti-inflammatory medicine, Vancomycin an antibiotic and finally ventilation. By the end of the pandemic, about one million Americans had died from Covid-19 according to CDC officials.

It's interesting to note that, I introduced Stabilized Allicin (a special garlic preparation) and IAG (inuloarabinogalactan, a special larch tree preparation), and before anyone even had a possible early treatment for Covid-19 in the United States. It's also interesting to note here that the Chinese were giving intravenous vitamin C to Covid-19 patients in body the ER and the ER waiting rooms at the exact time I was using my effective, lower cost treatment. The Chinese never did treat their people with an mRNA vaccine. You have to give those Chinese credit for taking better care of their people, even after being credited with accidentally or on purpose releasing this virus.

A year later, beginning in January 2021, our government at the urging of Fauci, allowed the toxic Ebola drug Remdesvir to become the first and only Covid-19 treatment drug for all of 2021. Fauci, his main assistant Birx and other government authorities certainly knew people were dying in the hospitals all throughout 2020 but ignored the need and the efforts by physicians to offer early treatment.

Fauci's course of action from the beginning of the pandemic has been to block early treatments of the Covid-19 disease. The verifiable truth is that our Anthony Fauci MD, the director of the National Institute of Allergy and Infectious Disease (NIAID), a government agency directly under the umbrella agency the National Institute of Health (NIH), worked diligently instead to **create** a dangerous pathogenic virus and give it to the Chinese. He had to do this because the Congress voted to stop him from continuing to bioengineer this virus. Fauci is being questioned right now by Congress as to whether this is true. He tries to deny it or just answers "I can't recall". He also refuses to give any documentation regarding the research done in 2020 to prove that the Covid-19 "vaccination" was tested for safety or its ability to prevent infection. The senate panel plans on continuing this investigation with more long days of examination of this now retired scientist.

Fauci waited while many of us got very sick and our loved ones died. Worse than that, he obtained approval for Remdesvir that along with other drugs and in the hospital killed fifty percent of those Covid patients that took it by destroying their kidneys. Those that survived the drugs met their demise from a ventilator at eight percent. Hospitals rarely ventilate serious Covid patients anymore, I wonder why?

It is a medical fact that the Covid-19 infection is different from the regular flu. When someone comes down with the regular flu, the hemoglobin molecule in their blood can still carry oxygen to all the various cells of the body. That is why more people survive the regular flu. Their brain, immune system and the rest of the body get the oxygen they need to fight the virus. However, the Covid-19 virus damages the hemoglobin in such a way that ventilators cannot work. If blood cannot carry oxygen because the hemoglobin is damaged, the chances of surviving a flu infection are very small.

Fauci's Remdesvir destroys kidney function by causing fluid to back up to the already compromised lungs by the virus. This fluid also puts pressure on the heart, which is partly why many patients died of cardiac complications in the ICU. As 2021 began, hospitals prescribed a triple mix of kidney destroying drugs for Covid-19 patients:

Remdesivir: destroys the kidneys of 35% of those who take it.

Vancomycin: destroys the kidneys of 10% of those who take it.

Dexamethasone: destroys the kidneys of 5% of those who take it.

Second grade math shows that this treatment will kill 50% percent of the kidneys of patients given this cocktail in the hospital ICU. In addition, as this treatment fails to help these patients survive the Covid-19 lung infection, the doctor finally puts them on a ventilator creating even more stress that according to CDC statistics kills eight percent of Covid-19 patients, eighty percent!

As 2020 proceeded, Fauci encouraged the persecution of physicians committed to early, outpatient treatment of Covid-19 patients. Later that year in the summer, physicians around the country offered other treatments than garlic and larch tree or other natural medicines. The first one was hydroxychloroquine. This began in June of 2020 when an ER physician used both hydroxychloroquine and zinc to cure 29 out of 30 patients who presented with Covid symptoms. Unfortunately, some peer reviewed studies over the next six months seem to suggest that hydroxychloroquine did not reduce mortality or morbidity of patients with Covid-19. Of course, these studies were apparently designed to disprove hydroxychloroquine's effectiveness because they ignored the ER physician's protocol by leaving out the zinc. When studies that used zinc were done and this protocol was shown to improve outcomes, physicians and patients began to gravitate back to it. Apparently, zinc allows the hydroxychloroquine to enter the virus directly and there is some evidence it helps repair the hemoglobin molecule so the patients can cure that way as well and carry oxygen more effectively.

In late 2020, Ivermectin came into the spotlight. This is a drug that had been used primarily for parasites originally derived from the hull of the black walnut. It was given to Covid-19 patients and then actively studied by various research organizations around the world. After more than eighteen peer-reviewed studies, it has become clear that Ivermectin is largely effective, especially if doxycycline was added to the treatment, at reducing symptoms and mortality of Covid-19.[13] [14]

13

You say you do not believe that Big Pharma cares more for their profits than your health? Then why didn't Fauci, the FTC, the hospitals, the doctors working there, the popular press and Joe Biden endorse, promote and repurpose a very safe drug like Ivermectin so that it could start saving lives in the last half of 2020 and all of 2021? Why did they not promote the use of hydroxychloroquine and zinc when Dr. Anthony Cardillo M.D. used it successfully with severe Covid patients in early 2020? Why did the research on hydroxychloroquine not include zinc when the mechanism of action was that hydroxychloroquine opens up the cell and the zinc flows in and stops replication of the virus? You cannot disprove

---

https://journals.lww.com/americantherapeutics/fulltext/2021/08000/ivermectin_for_prevention_and_treatment_of.7.aspx

14
https://www.ncbi.nlm.nih.gov/pmc/articles/PMC8088823/

treatment if you leave out a critical part of the protocol. Study them together or do not study them at all. Once the first study done on Covid-19 patients using hydroxychloroquine **alone** which showed no effect was completed the FDA withdrew the EUA (emergency use authorization).[15]

By August of 2020, a litany of physicians was complaining to Fauci about his refusal to keep the EUA for hydroxychloroquine available. Why did the government instead wait until January 2021 for the kidney-killing drug Remdesvir to be approved by the FDA?[16]

---

[15] https://abc7.com/coronavirus-covid-19-chloroquine-hydroxychloroquine/6082485/

[16] https://www.thedesertreview.com/opinion/columnists/open-letter-to-dr-anthony-fauci-regarding-the-use-of-hydroxychloroquine-for-treating-covid-19/article_31d37842-dd8f-11ea-80b5-bf80983bc072.html

In addition, what is worse our government has actively persecuted physicians encouraging the early treatment of Covid-19. For example: Peter McCullough M.D. and Sheri TenPenny D.O. were both censored by the American Board of Internal Medicine (ABIM), a new pro vaccine government agency that has the power to encourage state licensing boards to revoke a physician's license if the physician doesn't agree with their Covid-19 drug treatments and vaccine science. Apparently, government judges and prosecutors have abandoned the First Amendment. If a physician **dares to** disagree with the "State Religion of Medicine," they go after their livelihood by attacking their license because they have classified them as a "misinformation" doctor.[17]

---

[17] https://www.medpagetoday.com/special-reports/exclusives/101529

Chapter 3

My First Trial

It is August 2021 and seventeen months have passed since I was charged and indicted in May of 2020. The first trial will began and took an entire week. My attorneys brought in three witnesses who had benefited from the use of Stabilized Allicin and IAG when they were down with Covid-19 symptoms. The prosecutor flew FDA agents in from Washington D.C. and Oakland California. There were over 100 Affidavits from my patients handed in to the courts but these were not allowed by the judge to be available for the jury to deliberate with. The prosecutor complained that I stated my products could "cure" Covid-19. These Affidavits confirmed that I had never said that Stabilized Allicin would cure any disease especially Covid-19. I merely exercised my First Amendment right to inform people that these products could treat or prevent ANY infection from the long lived experience of countless physicians across the world, clinic studies done in various venues and even controlled "laboratory" studies available in the National Library of Medicine. My attorneys also brought this point up on the record. Score one point for me exercising my First Amendment right of free speech to express my opinion that these products could be used to reduce infections no matter what microorganism was associated with whatever disease a patient was challenged with including viruses like Covid-19 and boost the immune system to finish the job.

When the prosecutor complained about my continuing to use my naturopathic credential ND, while "legally" practicing as a health coach, The Washington D.C. senior FDA witness rebuffed the man saying…"Even though Dr. Marschall does not have a current license, he received his credential from an accredited naturopathic institution. He can continue to use his ND credential." Score a second point for me. The interesting thing here to me was, twelve years ago I stood in front of the second trial judge, Judge Settle in Federal Court for a different issue and the prosecutor at the time asked the judge to order me NOT to use my credential while I was suspended. That suspension lasted two years and allowed me to practice as if nothing had ever happened. The judge said into the public record that very thing, that I received my credential from a private medical school and therefore no prosecutor or even the state of Washington Department of Health could ever stop me from using my credential. My credential has and will always be out of any legal jurisdiction. Only a medical license lies within the jurisdiction of a state's department of health.

Then the Oakland FDA agent took the stand. The FDA had used this woman to lie to me and make a purchase of the two products. This entrapment was in a sense how it all started. It occurred in March of 2020. After she was sworn in the prosecutor played a 25-minute recording of our conversation and then a twenty-minute recording that occurred the next day. During these recordings, the jury learned that this agent told me she was in my wife's Facebook group and had heard good things about the treatment. She pretended she was a single mom who was afraid of Covid-19 affecting her two daughters especially although she admitted neither she nor her children were currently sick. Over the course of the two recordings I asked her questions about her health and encouraged her to consider dietary changes. I also encouraged her to take simple inexpensive nutritional supplements like vitamin D and vitamin C as preventative medicine since she was a single mom on a limited income. I held back on encouraging her to make a purchase because these two products are generally used to treat Covid-19, not to prevent it and the price at the time was $120 for both because the cost of importing it from Europe was high.

"Oh, no she remonstrated; I really want you to send them to me." You see, without getting me to send her the products, the FDA wouldn't have jurisdiction because they can ONLY charge someone if the person is shipping across state lines since they are a federal agency. The state of Washington while having the authority to charge me if I had harmed someone, had no authority to do more than investigate a complaint by an individual in Washington. To be clear, this was the real reason the case against my early treatment of Covid-19 began. A woman noticed a Facebook entry my wife posted that described her reversal of Covid-19 symptoms from consuming these two substances. This woman and another man here in our home town area of Sequim and Port Angeles, Washington, considered anyone promoting early natural treatment for Covid-19 to be dangerous. The both complained about this social media information to the Washington State Department of Health who had no interest in investigating me as there had been no complaints of harm, just these two good citizens watching out for dangerous people like me encouraging people to try a non-invasive, non-toxic plant based approach rather than go to the hospital where many simply died of a lack of really ANY rational approach to proper treatment.

I told this lying FDA sting operator that I would send the two products but to just leave them on the shelf and if she or her daughters came down with Covid-19 symptoms then she would have a treatment and to use it according to the directions that came with the box.

My attorney asked her "So is it a fact that you lied to my client to get him to ship his nutritional supplement across state lines?" She responded yes. This was entrapment, deliberate, clear and unconstitutional. Score a third point for me as the constitution the inviolable contract all Americans have with their federal government.

On cross-examination my attorney asked her about the FDA statute that I was charged with, keeping in mind that a statute is not a **law.** He read from the 21 USC 331 statute, the section the prosecutor was using to charge me with, "entering into interstate commerce a drug that is intended to prevent, mitigate or cure any disease." Now he was ready to attack the substance of the prosecutor's arguments. He asked the FDA agent "Are garlic capsules drugs? She said, "No they're nutritional supplements". The prosecutor interjected here that "it doesn't matter that garlic is a nutritional supplement, the fact that both on the recording and from the scientific evidence that came with the package suggesting that garlic is antiviral, it's enough to satisfy the statute and lead to a conviction."

Next came the most ridiculous part of the trial in my opinion. My attorney came back to the FDA agent with, "So, if my elderly grandmother sends me a birthday cake and says it could cheer me up would that qualify as a felony according to 21 USC 331?" "She thought for a few seconds and reluctantly replied…yes it would." Score a fourth point for me as my attorney was getting down to nitty-gritty of the case against me which defied common sense and there for the constitutionality of the statute.

Statutes are "guidelines" not laws. An FDA statute allows this federal agency to prosecute a U.S. citizen if there is evidence that harm to another citizen occurred. A statute does not allow the FDA to go on a witch-hunt. There is nothing in the U.S. Constitution that prevents any American from saying that garlic can prevent or treat viruses. The fact that there is substantial evidence, as you shall soon see that garlic and larch starch are very effective at treating a virus, especially Covid-19 is completely irrelevant to prosecutors. They seem to have one job and one job only. Protect the Big Pharma's lock on the economic control of the treatment of disease in this country.

The trial began on Monday and by Friday, two members of the jury had decided I had the right under the Constitution's First Amendment to say anything I wanted about garlic or anything else. They stood up for me and every business in the United States to sell garlic across state lines which is also legal under the Constitution. Therefore, this trial ended in a "mistrial". I was not acquitted but I was not guilty, as all twelve members had to agree with the prosecutor's arguments to convict. Score a fifth and final point to me, only because two common sense souls spoke up against the other 10 wrong thinking jurors and spoke the truth.

The first trial is over but at this point, this first judge decided to defy the Constitution by ignoring the establishment and intention of the seventh Amendment: "In Suits at common law, where the value in controversy shall exceed twenty dollars, the right of trial by jury shall be preserved, and no fact tried by a jury, shall be otherwise re-examined in any Court of the United States, then according to the rules of the common law."

This judge defied the usual comportment of a Federal District Court judge. He told the jury, "**In general prosecutors and defending lawyers are not allowed to talk with jurors after a trial. Regardless I am going to allow that to occur for this trial now.** After you leave the courtroom, while you're out in the hallway, I'd like you to stay behind so the prosecutor can ask you some questions." Really!

Just like that, the prosecutor asked the jurors in the outer hallway, **after** the trial was over, a series of questions that gave him insight into how to conspire with the next judge to craft different jury instructions to acquire a conviction at a new trial. This appeared to me to be more corruption by the federal government, presumably to protect Big Pharma, more obfuscation of the law of the land. My attorneys, my wife, my children and witnesses that appeared in my defense were shocked and exasperated at the appalling lack of justice and due process.

The next trial was two months later in October of 2021. During that time, one of the jurors that stood up against the loss of my constitutional rights called me and said he had purchased the two products. He wanted me to know how sorry he felt that I was treated so unlawfully and poorly by our own government.

Chapter 4

My Second Trial

By now two more months had passed. I hope none of my readers will ever have to go through a prolonged legal battle with their own government. The worst part of this experience is the waiting. These thoughtless, careless, unscrupulous judicial operatives of our country's agencies and courts are quite willing to put anyone they set their sights on through long-term mental and emotional stress. It does not seem to matter to them that no "harm is done", it matters not at all that there is no "cause of action". They act above the law and step on whomever they want to. Every night during this ordeal, I went to bed wondering when the next action will take place and whether or not they were going to take my personal freedom away.

During this trial, a professor of Botanical Medicine from Bastyr University took the stand. He spoke straight to the jury and for the next 25 minutes explained the history and studies showing the clinical effectiveness of both allicin and larch. He was quite clear that there had even been placebo-controlled studies on the use of **allicin in cases of Covid-19**, which showed allicin was quite effective in reducing symptoms and saving lives.

My attorneys brought some of my people to the stand to give their testimony to this new jury. One witness flew up all the way from Arizona. A tactic my attorney explained was used to show solidarity with my Constitutional right to ship him these products across state lines.

The prosecutor brought the original FDA entrapment agent from Oakland California and we had to sit through the same recordings and testimony for this new jury. Again, when asked by my attorney about his grandmother and birthday cake, she gave the same answer, "yes, your grandmother would be guilty of violating 21 USC 331". It was interesting to me that this time the prosecutor did not intervene. He had seemed quite laid back at this second trial and I was soon to know why.

On Thursday, the jurors were given instructions by the judge. First, he told them very clearly, "**you are not to consider the Constitution in your deliberations**". Excuse me? We are in a federal court and a judge, sworn to uphold the Constitution, is telling a jury of my peers that they cannot talk with each other about the United States Constitution? Are you shocked? My wife, my children and I, all sitting in the courtroom are looking at each other and simply could not believe what we were hearing! Why have a U.S. Constitution if when you get to a federal court, the judge sits there and tells the jury, "Hey, forget about the constitution, it's not important, just do what I tell you to do". Second, the judge tells the jury, "You are not to consider the scientific evidence presented by the professor from the naturopathic medical school. You are to ignore any evidence presented regarding of the effectiveness of the garlic extract with Covid-19 patients". Wow judge! The defense brings forth evidence that you and the prosecutor does not like, and you demand the jury ignore it? Now if I had been in an Australian courtroom, and there were kangaroos all around, I would not have been surprised. Instead, I was in America where, when a judge allows a witness to spend twenty minutes explaining the science of garlic and infections to a jury without the judge stopping this witness and informing the jury that his evidence is inadmissible, he does not get to take that evidence away from them just before their deliberations, just because he feels like it. This is **not** due process.

Then he went on to tell the jury the only three things they were allowed to consider:

1. Did he sell a drug across state lines?
2. Did he prescribe a drug across state lines?

3. Did he say this drug could prevent, mitigate, treat or cure a disease?

Oh, and of course he reminded them not to discuss the constitution. He did not want that ridiculous document to get in the prosecutors' way of a conviction, after all, the government had already spent over **1.5 million dollars** on this case and it would be an embarrassment to the government if the jury acquitted me.

On Friday morning, the jury came back with the following:

1. No, he did not sell a drug across state lines because garlic and larch are nutritional supplements not drugs.
2. No, he did not prescribe a drug across state lines because garlic and larch are nutrition supplements not drugs.
3. Yes, he did say it could prevent, mitigate or treat a disease.

The FDA statute tried to make a nutritional supplement into a drug when it is not a drug and the jury, who cannot consider the Constitution now has to answer questions on a form only, no relevant discussion because the Constitution is out of the picture. The judge advises them that if they answer yes to any one of the questions that I will be convicted. The prosecutor and the judge created this form in such a way as to achieve a specific result, a sort of 'fill in the blanks' conviction. The entire jury came back with the opinion that garlic and larch are nutritional supplements. As you can see from their answers to questions one and two, they were not buying it that these natural medicines are drugs. But question three was worded, thanks to the first judge allowing the prosecutor to question the jury AFTER the trial, so they could only answer yes to number three. Sure, the constitution allows people to give their opinions about natural products but the jury was ordered to ignore that famous document.

What could have happened if the judge had allowed the jury to consider the constitution? Well, the First Amendment allows freedom of speech. Any American can go around saying garlic can help an infection even across state lines. We are talking about nutritional supplements and free speech by lay people such as me. The FDA has no jurisdiction over lay people who say chicken soup can help a cold or the flu let alone garlic and larch.

What could have happened if the judge had allowed the jury to consider the evidence that garlic can help with Covid-19 symptoms? This information would have allowed the jury even more confidence that I spoke the truth when I said garlic could help with viruses, even the Covid-19 virus. Not that they even needed that evidence. I was not on trial for harming anyone. There was no lawsuit against me by an injured party. No one who had ever purchased my garlic or larch tree starch product suffered serious side effects. No one had died after taking them either. Many people have died after going to the emergency room at thousands of hospitals all across the country complaining of Covid-19 symptoms.

Chapter 5

My Sentence

More waiting, I hate waiting. It's now 5 months later in March of 2022 and the judge looks me straight in the eye for the first time and delivers his sentence. "Mr. Marschall, you are a dangerous man for offering an alternative treatment at the beginning of the pandemic, instead of waiting for the government to approve a treatment for Covid-19." Note that Anthony Fauci had already approved Remdesvir in January the year before and we know how that worked out. Also, at the same time the so called 'Covid-19 vaccine' was released and we're certainly finding out how that's working out. "I sentence you to 8 months in a federal prison".

Ouch! No more waiting at least, now I have an answer but eight months! It is interesting to note that his own probation department officers had advised him of three possible sentence options: no jail time, supervised release or 6 months prison time at the most. He added 2 months to their suggestions. What an outstanding protector of the peace he was.

So help me out here, at the beginning of the pandemic, if you knew of a nutritional supplement, not birthday cake, that had been effective against the flu in the past, would you have offered it to your grandmother? Do you believe The Constitution's First Amendment should protect your right to speak about a nutritional supplement against unscrupulous prosecutors who set up entrapment schemes and acrimonious judges who do not follow the constitution? Even if you chose to wait until January to receive Remdesvir or get your Covid-19 vaccine, do you think anyone else who wanted early treatment should have been denied that option? I was simply low hanging fruit for an FDA prosecutor trolling for an alternative physician to sacrifice on the altar of Big Pharma to further his career when Covid-19 showed up.

Chapter 6

Prelude to Prison

I was scheduled to enter Camp Sheridan, a federal prison in Sheridan, Oregon, an hour south of Portland on June 27, 2022. My birthday is June 22nd. I was a little preoccupied with going to prison so when my wife encouraged me to come with her to a vegan cooking class at a local church the day before my birthday, I was quite surprised to be greeted by 50 people including some of my children and my classic rock band. The band had snuck the equipment out of the rehearsal studio that day without me seeing them and Rose had organized all the food and the people without me ever realizing what was going on.

Seeing the support of all those people really helped me go to prison with a positive feeling. It meant a lot. Five days later Rose drove me to Sheridan and I 'voluntarily surrendered' to the Federal Bureau of Prisons.

Chapter 7

Solitary Confinement

When I got to the 100 acre Federal Prison Complex in Sheridan, Oregon I walked into the Detention Center which is where all convicted men must first report before they are directed to either the prison cells in the Detention Center itself, the prison cells of the Medium Prison or the open dormitory like wings of the Prison Camp.

The medical correction officers who did the intake of new inmates asked me if I had been vaccinated for Covid and if so to show them a credential as proof. After responding that I had not been vaccinated I was administered a nasal swab for Covid-19 and told I was negative which of course means I did not have the virus. After further examination the medical officer said I did not appear to have any symptoms of Covid-19 or symptoms of any illness but regardless he was required to immediately put into solitary confinement for ten days.

The experience I will next relate was the most egregious thing that has ever happened to me and the most upsetting experience in my seventy two years of life. When I first began writing this book I decided not to mention it because it was too painful to recount. Eventually my editor, friends and family encouraged me to tell this as part of the whole story.

They called this ten day pre-federal prison camp detour, "isolation". I was placed in a six by ten foot cell that had a bunk bed with only one thin mattress (this will be important later), dressed in orange pants and a V-neck shirt. I was also issued a jacket, two sheets and one thin blanket.

By the time I was introduced to my Spartan accommodations, it was lunch time. They actually read my intake form, realized I was a vegan and at 1pm slid a peanut butter and jelly sandwich on white bread and an apple through the slot in the door.

I spent the afternoon and early evening walking back and forth, attempting unsuccessfully to wear out the linoleum. Dinner arrived again through the slot, a tasteful serving of ramen which I chose to decline because it was soaked in chicken broth. I chose to water fast instead and hope for better fair at a later date.

That evening, I made the bed with my bottom, top sheet and the paper thin blanket. After I got into bed I realized the thin mattress had compressed down to a half inch over a sheet of steel and. I had the choice of adding the jacket as a second layer of insulation or using it as a pillow. Since I have a neck injury from age sixteen, I had to use the jacket as a pillow since I can only sleep on my side.

I was kept there all day without being able to leave the cell. The vent in the ceiling was constantly blowing cold air at my head. I slept in the same space I urinated and defecated. The room was poorly lit. The walls were cinder block construction but the overhead vents transmitted dull cacophonies of the fifty inmates that were allowed to walk the indoor track, play cards or games in the downstairs dayroom or go outside every day into a yard for exercise or basketball.

Not me though no, I did my stretching routine about every hour. I sang songs from my rather large collection to keep sane. There was only the hard bunk bed, no chair so I couldn't meditate sitting on the bed as my legs won't go into a full or even half lotus anymore and the bed was like a rock anyway. There was also a hard steel bunk bed frame above my head so sitting would have compressed my spine as well.

My cold, barren metal frame was so hard I tossed and turned all night long. I have some arthritis in both shoulders from sleeping on them only for 55 years since my neck fracture, never being able to get comfortable on my stomach or back. If you've ever been awake without even once drifting off to sleep for an entire seventy-two hours, you'll probably experience the mental aberration I did whereby you want desperately to stop your mind from thinking, hoping each moment that you will drift off. I sincerely hope I never experience that again because it's as close to what I imagine it's like for people who find they are going insane.

The shoulder, back and hip pain got to be intolerable, more so than even the isolation. My room had a large vent that constantly blew cold air. It was literally aimed directly at the bed and never stopped, day or night. The cold was really bad, especially at night when the body temperature drops down anyway. I just couldn't sleep in all that coldness and pain.

At the end of the third day I was convinced that I was in enough pain, chill and high anxiety from the lack of sleep that I would be dead soon. That was when things began to change. An inmate the morning of the fourth day managed to fold a book in half and squeeze it under my door. Now I had something to help distract my mind from the cold, pain and sleep deprivation. Then finally latter that day a correction officer gave me an additional blanket so the cold, air conditioned air stopped putting me into hypothermia. That was also the day they let me have a shower. They put everyone, about fifty inmates, into their cells and let me have thirty minutes to find the shower, use it, dry off and get back to my cell.

So I wasn't going to die, well that was promising. But now I was concerned about the worry Rose would be going through. I couldn't communicate with my wife or ANYONE outside my cell, not even other inmates as they walked by my cell door. I was sure she would have tried to contact me and since that didn't have the consideration to communicate to her on my behalf I could only wait until this was all over.

A correction officer on day eight in the evening when I was able to take my second shower tried to help me get on a computer to contact Rose. It didn't work. She never ended up finding out about my ordeal until I was transferred to the camp on day eleven.

At the end of the ten days of confinement they let me out. By the way, when I got to the camp that day, every other person I spoke with that was put into solitary confinement, had spent only five days there. Kind of makes you wonder huh? As I was led through the labyrinthine corridors of the detention center I noticed I stopped shivering and was able to walk more erect as I got closer to seeing the warm sun through the large windows of the lobby. Without anything more than a, "Go that way to the camp" by a correction officer, I was then allowed to walk downhill about 300 feet by myself from the Detention Center building where my solitary confinement cell had been located to Camp Sheridan.

Chapter 8

Prison

The federal prison known as Camp Sheridan is for non-violent offenders. The reason I was able to saunter down from the federal detention center to the federal prison camp was that the prison camp had a few barriers but no walls. Had I chosen, I could have walked into the nearby town of Sheridan and from there travelled to go to other locations. The fences around the camp were at the north end and only constructed to keep the town of Sheridan residents from venturing into the federal prison by accident or design.

Remember we're discussing a hundred acres that simply allowed any inmate to leave at any time. Unfortunately, if they did so without approval, they would be sent to a walled-in facility for a period of time, like the federal detention center I had just left, but generally to Nevada or even California federal prisons because the system took you farther away to make an impression on you that you had not only lost your camp openness but your local connections. In the event that a camp inmate should leave, although he wouldn't get more time added to his sentence he would temporality be denied the freedoms he had enjoyed in the camp. Approval to leave was rare anyway from what I learned later. You could ask for a 'furlough' which allowed an inmate to leave for up to 10 days for a funeral or birth or special medical procedure but furloughs were almost never granted for absolutely no other reason that for the warden to be unreasonable.

There were about 240 inmates when I arrived. To be in a federal prison camp for a newbie you cannot have ever been convicted of physically harming anyone. If you came into the camp from a walled prison like the Federal Medium prison which housed violent offenders, you would have had to have been observed by the correction officers at the

Medium there as having changed your ways for often a year or more that you could be allowed to finish your sentence at the Camp. I didn't meet many of those.

The inmates in the camp are there basically for 2 different reasons, white collar crime or drug sales; some people believe, especially illegal drug salespeople that drug sales is a white collar crime when committed by non-violent offenders, You'll have to decide that one for yourself. The drug dealer numbers were at about eighty percent leaving about twenty percent inmates convicted of white collar crimes like me.

The drug dealing ranged from marijuana, to cocaine, meth, heroin and fentanyl. It was easy to spot the meth dealers, most of them had no teeth and you had a hard time understanding what they were saying even if they had some in their mouth.

The white collar inmates were there mostly for income tax evasion, Income tax avoidance is legal, the government lets you or your tax accountant uncover deductions you are legally allowed. This is opposed to evading taxes by just not paying them or using the US Constitution and the 16th amendment to try to convince the IRS you never had to in the first place.

There was one inmate in the camp that had actually written a book on the reasons he didn't pay his income taxes. The information was quite interesting and basically produced evidence that federal income tax has always been voluntary. But there he was so does it really matter if some old dusty document like the 1789 US Constitution or the 1933 16th Amendment can be interpreted to mean taxes are voluntary when the IRS agents, the collection agents for the US Treasury ignore such a notion? Ask Wesley Snipes who spent three years in a Federal Camp for his beliefs about personal income taxes.

There were some others convicted of unusual white collar crimes ranging from fraudulent investment impropiaties to real estate fraud. I met a dentist there who had been at the camp for 8 years of a 10 year sentence. He told me his story in the cafeteria when I first arrived. He started with his long career that had eventually listed him in some GQ kind of magazine as one of the top 100 dentists in the United States. He worked in a busy city in California caring for the entire UPS drivers and staff. His office manager he reported to me after a few years started skimming off his books in such a clever way that he didn't notice. She accumulated quite a small fortune after ten years such that he couldn't help but notice. He said he went to the local police detectives asking them for help dealing with this fraud. The detectives advised him that they wouldn't intervene to help him get her charged with fraud. On the other hand, she started to get wind that her boss knew of her crime and DID get the police to intervene by accusing this dentist with overcharging UPS to get the attention off her crime. The interesting thing was, after he had been imprisoned for 4 years, police investigations DID find her culpable but never used this evidence to exonerate him!

I was put in a "cube" in a dormitory in one of two buildings, each having four wings. The building was built like an X and had two stories. Each cube held a maximum of six beds and each cube was only separated from the one next to it by a five food high cinda block wall. There was a hall separating each set of four cubes. I was given three pairs of "greens", only Camp inmates get that color. Orange is for Federal Detention Centers like when I was in solitary confinement, Federal Medium prisons and Federal Maximum prisons. The greens were quite sturdy pants and shirts and had to be worn into the cafeteria at breakfast and lunch. At dinner and after 4 pm you could wear gray sweatpants and sweatshirts purchased from the commissary. The socks and underwear were another matter; the ones they gave you for free were worn out, stiff and scratchy. I am so glad that my dear Rose had put money in my account before I even got there so I could order some decent socks and briefs.

It was very hot in early July when I arrived at the Camp. Being under the Federal Bureau of Prisons (BOP) your life while there is supposed to be regulated by the Congress. When I got there, a Congressional Law called the First Step Act of 2018 was in place to allow the wardens in the United States prisons to allow "good time" for early release if the inmate complied with certain requirements. Every inmate had a "case manager" who gave him a "computed release date" document early in his confinement. My document said I had to attend two classes, work at a job, and not receive any "shots" before I could be released to a halfway house. A shot is when you disobey any rules the BOP has in regards to certain behaviors:

- Taking food from the cafeteria
- Leaving the cube during a "count"
- Vaping or smoking a cigarette
- Using a cell phone

- Receiving contraband from an outside friend or family member

Chapter 9

Horticulture

Before I begin describing my work at the camp, it will be interesting for the reader to know that a large proportion of the 240 inmates had jobs. There were some disabled guys that couldn't work, usually the three guys in wheelchairs but others had disabilities that were not visible and there weren't quite enough jobs anyway. The big picture though is that camp inmates did ALL the jobs for the entire 100 acre Federal prison camp which included the Detention center, the Medium prison and the camp. It took just a few correctional officers, (CO's) to organize about 200 camp inmates to work in

Electrical, Plumbing, Agriculture, Horticulture, Construction, Cafeteria and other functions for all three parts of the entire prison which housed about 1,600 souls.

I was very fortunate to get a job in the Horticulture department about a half a mile away from my building. Camp Sheridan is a campus of about 20 acres with classrooms, a chapel, a cafeteria, a phone area, an administration office, 2 dormitories, a quarter mile track, a baseball diamond, a recreation area with weights, outdoor basketball courts, handball courts and pickleball courts. Each dormitory wing had its own bathroom and TV room. The TV rooms were designated by race. Apparently that policy evolved from the inmates themselves, why I'm not sure but then I'm not racist, I get along well with everyone, well, everyone except FDA federal prosecutors and judges.

My job in the Horticulture department was a real Godsend. No question. I love to work outdoors, to garden, I had even taught organic gardening to my classmates when I was premed at California State University in San Jose back in the day. Rose and I have had a garden every year we've been together going on 46 years now.

In my cube, one of the "campers" as I liked to call the inmates was a friendly black man I will call George who is about my age and began working with me from the start. We would walk over to the Horticulture area about 7 am and do whatever we were told. At first it was removing drip irrigation hoses from areas that had been harvested. Next it was weeding the extensive flower gardens in front of the greenhouses that took most of July. It was hot, sweaty work but we enjoyed both the outdoor aspect and getting tanned and strong.

The Horticulture area is about 10 acres and consists of two 100 foot long and 30 foot wide greenhouses surrounded by soil beds for vegetables, flower gardens, orchards, compost piles and irrigation canals with small Japanese garden style bridges.

There are many shade trees all around the horticulture acres in this flat valley surrounded by low lying hills.

In August, watering flowers around the entire 100-acre complex which included the Federal Medium Prison, the Federal Detention Center and The Federal Prison Camp, a job maintained by the Horticulture department came open. George and I were told to get with the outgoing driver and learn the ropes. The current driver I will call Paul was a friendly guy who, to begin, drove us around the place in a Kawasaki "Mule", a vehicle that looks like a utilitarian golf cart, pointing out the various buildings so we had the big picture of where we would be working.

Watering consisted initially of filling a 100-gallon metal box that sat in the mule, adding pressure to it from a compressor at the campus garage and driving anywhere there were hanging flower pots or flower boxes and watering with a hose from this box or a prefilled 6-gallon watering can. Eventually, the pressurized metal box was deemed unsafe by the CO so we stuck to longs hoses and watering cans.

Due east of Horticulture is the Federal Correctional Institution also known as the "Medium". This facility houses the "middle" violent offenders. There are more of these prisons in the Federal system than any other type. In a Medium you wear orange and you live in a cell with occasional chances to exercise in a yard for an hour.

Working in horticulture was almost every inmates preference compared to kitchen food preparation, serving food or any janitorial work. Electricians, plumbers, mechanics, and carpenters had electric mules so they had more interesting experiences but they were a small group. In horticulture you had the entire 100 acre camp as your workspace and a greater variety of projects and learning experiences that could serve you when you were released.

Watering the hanging flower pots, the long boxed flowers and other flower beds was a more sophisticated procedure than you might at first imagine. When George and I took over the duties of our soon to be released predecessor, we had a one hundred gallon rectangular metal tank sitting in the mule truck bed to be able to reach flowers that were very distant from horticulture. We would fill it up each morning to the eighty percent mark and then pressurize it with air from the nearby prison garage where the mechanics took care of the prison vehicles. Our first stop was the one and only entrance to the one hundred acre complex that had a large flower bed sitting in front of the eight by 6 "Camp Sheridan, Federal Prison Complex" sign. This entrance came from a county road with farmland as far as you could see on either side. We would park the mule in front of the sign, run the hose to the flower beds and release the water to feed petunias, marigolds, cactus and other flowers and bushes. Next we went to the "White House". This building was situated a half a mile on the main prison road from the entrance and three hundred feet from the Administrative building of the camp.

This was the training facility for the correction officers. It had a two story house with bedrooms, kitchen, bathrooms and such. Right next to it were educational rooms. It was called the white house only by the camp inmates, mainly because it was painted bright white and, well, it was a federal government building after all. The flowers and bushes along the walkways in front of the training building were quite extensive. Sometimes during our routine watering we would hear rock and roll coming from the center but mostly it was quiet. On one occasion the entire horticulture department, about 20 guys, came out to complete a major overhaul of the vegetation surrounding the "White House". This included trimming hedges in the back that bordered a river. The river ran all along the north border of the Sheridan Federal Prison Complex and represented a kind of northern moat for the prison. We would occasionally see a fishing boat trolling the waters but not often. The city of Sheridan was a pretty small town and even a few onlookers at our prison were rare.

After leaving the "White House" in our mule we went to the Detention Center where I did my 10 days of "solitary confinement". The walkway up to the door was surrounding by elaborate flower beds with boxed flowers closed to the front door. So many different flowers and hanging pots dotted the walkway it took quite a lot of water to soak it up in the hot August sun.

We next turned around and crossed the main prison road and water an even more extensive flower bed directly in front of the administrative building. The administrative building included a large multi-purpose room on the right for inmate meetings and visitation. The offices to the left were for the senior guards, the medical clinic and the dental office. Flowers in August were just beautiful and all the buildings had hanging pots. Petunias, pansies, marigolds, nasturtiums, you name it we had it. My point here is that, the Federal government takes care of its own. Whether you might imagine this botanical dressing of the complex was more for the camp inmates who were the most free and therefore allowed to enjoy the grounds or it was really more for the correction officers to help assuage the stress of them being around the prisoners, you'll have to make up your mind about yourself.

After leaving the camp Administrative building, we turned south on the main prison complex road, passing the ten acre camp, the ten acre horticulture complex, the service buildings (carpentry, mechanic garage, electrical engineer and plumbing) and went to the very southern border to the Federal Medium prison, the largest building in the complex. We parked on the road in front of the entrance and watered even more earthen beds, boxed flowers and hanging pots. George and I worked very well together. He was an affable sort, a guy with a big smiles and an easy temperament. He was a retired heavy equipment operator and as happy as I to be winging around in this mule, breathing fresh air and assimilating the beauty of the flowers and the surrounding hills of middle Oregon.

On day, about 5 weeks into our watering career, while watering the beds in front of the medium, a correction officer came storming out of the door and spoke harshly to me about his issue. I had never seen him before, spoke with him or had really anything to do with ANY medium anybody. He complained that our watering predecessor had failed to give him the name of a particular beautiful flower in the beds on the road in front of the entrance. He seemed so angry that I just stood there trying to think of how I could scale this confrontation down without winding up in the medium myself. I apologized for the lack of follow-up of my "colleague" and promised to get him the information he needed about the flower the very next day. This seemed to mollify him but he left with this enjoinder, "I know people in your camp, if you don't get me the common and Latin name of this plant by tomorrow, I will have to find you a bed inside here". Well, you can imagine my anxiety and my efforts next to get him those names before I came back the following day.

Finally we turned around and went to our last responsibility, the camp itself. Our job here was extensive: water ALL the hanging flower pots everywhere, in front of the dormitories, the chapel and the hallways. The hallways included the dental office, the medical office, the inner door to the administrative offices, the barber shop, the room with the bank of five landline phones and chairs campers used to call out to family and friends, the laundry, the commissary where we purchased products, the cafeteria, the horticulture classroom, the library, the computer classroom, three general classrooms, the physical education office, the gymnasium and the sports office. This long continuous string of places was one quarter mile long. I knew that because when it rained and I couldn't walk the regulation quarter mile track in the general recreation area, I walked this one continuous hallway which took me just as long as one walk around the track.

Horticulture workers were sort of celebrities amongst the other campers. When we showed up in our mule, people stepped aside and often spoke with us about our travels around the hundred acres and our experiences. Although technically, any inmate could travel past the ten acres of the camp, if you're were caught outside camp grounds you were often a "shot", a mark against your good record. More on that later. So, inmates had to rely on us for a bigger view of the happenings out there on the entire one hundred acre complex.

At the beginning of September, my last month, the one hundred gallon metal tank on the mule sprung a leak. We drove it over to welding shop and they did their best to repair it. Unfortunately, the correctional officer in charge didn't like the look of the welds so to be safe he said, we would have to carry hundred foot long hoses and watering buckets to do our work. The flowers were expected to start dying out by October first so we only to water for a few weeks longer anyway.

Chapter 10

The Big Treat

At the end of July, the blackberries were in bloom and ready to be picked. When this happens every year the inmate who is head of Horticulture, a man I will call Adam, lets the Horticulture staff know about a special project. The project is to pick enough blackberries to feed blackberry cobbler to the approximately 300 inmates in the camp and about 200 inmates in the Detention Center. Not the blackberries on the ten-acre Horticulture campus. We had only two fifty foot rows of berries on our property because the Horticulture department was a vocational training program. There were always two classes with about ten students each learning principles of plant biology, agriculture and hydroponics with field trips to the facility.

Whatever food we grew in the soil or the hydroponic greenhouse was available to the students and the workers only. We were strictly forbidden to sell food to campers.

At the very southeast part of the 100-acre complex, up on a hill overlooking acres of farmland was a huge blackberry patch over 500 feet long. The students and the Horticulture staff spent two days picking blackberries enough to make a cobbler prepared by a Horticulture worker I will call Wilhelm, who in real life was also a chef and owner of several restaurants. It was hard but fun work. We had with us boards that were twelve inches wide by two inches deep and twelve feet long. When we picked all the low hanging fruit we laid the boards across the bushes to get at the berries way in the back. It was a "teeter-totter" experience that taught me just how high and close we were to the ridge overlooking the farmland. At one point I crept up to the edge of the board overlooking the rural area within six inches of a 100-foot drop. I'm sure the stickers would have stopped my fall but I was lucky enough to never find out.

We were outside in the warm sun, doing something that made you feel like a normal person in your own community and what's more we got to help feed others who rarely got such a tasty natural treat. Later on I learned that Adam had been required to spend three days contacting several different offices at the facility getting permission for us to do this. I also learned that Liam had spent many hours baking huge cobblers for over 500 inmates.

Chapter 11

Ryan

Ryan was the official director of the Horticulture department. He delegated responsibilities to three other senior staff, gave out the orders to the rest of us, and organized the calendar and purchases of equipment, seeds and anything else we needed. He had more knowledge about the overall workings of the entire Bureau of Prisons as well as the Horticulture department than anyone I ever met and became a kind of mentor to me. If I didn't understand something that was occurring or might affect me, I waited until I heard his explanation before I felt comfortable with an answer. I learned about the First Step Act from him. He was keen to understand it as it was even more important for him to know so he could help others get a sense of when they could theoretically get released.

As an example, although he knew well that the warden didn't consistently honor the First Step Act, he knew it enough that before my case manager had figured out my "elderly offender release date," he was able to tell me exactly when I should be released: December 6th, five months and eleven days from entering the Camp, released after serving two-thirds of my eight month sentence. He explained that to me after I had been at the Camp only two weeks while the case manager took three months to give me the same answer.

The First Step act he explained was a Congressional Act passed in 2018 to provide for the early release of inmates who showed good efforts to abide by BOP requirements. Unfortunately, this act has not been properly implemented to date. Very few inmates had been released according to their opportunities for early release for "good time". The guys I worked with within Horticulture were all convicted of the so-called white collar crime. These were smart guys in their middle ages mostly. With Ryan's help they read and complied with the rules and requirements of the First Step Act yet one-by-one, they were refused release by a criminally negligent warden.

One camper had been there for over three months before he was finally released to a halfway house. Another was given a release date document and a copy of a bus ticket but at the last minute was told his case manager hadn't done the release paperwork properly so he wouldn't get out for twelve more days. The next case was the absolute worst of all.

Chapter 12

Wilhelm

My closest friend in Horticulture was Wilhelm. He was the hardest working and most skilled soil gardener of us all. He was in charge of the second greenhouse, the soil greenhouse. He grew many kinds of seedlings there and then transplanted them out into the soil when they got big enough. He was very vigilant about his work. He wanted the work done right and as long as you were careful to do it his way there was harmony on the farm. His wife was a horticulturalist on the outside and he had learned quite a bit from her experience. I'll never forget when I was first given my position in horticulture of how beautiful and orderly his outside beds were. They were positioned immediately next to the two greenhouses facing the flower gardens to the north. Next to the acre of vegetable plants was another acre of apple and pear trees. South of that were rows of blueberries, grown by the students. Going further south there were rows of tomatillos. To the east of those were more flower beds. In the middle of these various gardens was an experimental garden. It was completely fenced in and contained a very large collection of vegetable plants and fruit plans. The story I got about this garden was that someone a while back believed if you mixed fruits and vegetables in close proximity through more active bee pollination you would succeed in achieving a higher crop yield.

At the beginning of August, our main inmate steward Ryan decided it was time to wake up the hydroponic greenhouse. So, on top of our flower watering duties, we spent time in a very warm three thousand square foot greenhouse. The first day I began working there, I got so hot that I took off my shirt and worked bare-chested. When Ryan came in he looked at me, closed his eyes and said, "You know Garlic Rick, that's something I will never be able to un-see". I was pretty sure I wasn't "that" ugly bare-chested but regardless, I cut off the sleeves of an undershirt, put on this makeshift tank top and learned to live with the hundred and five degree temperature.

My job in the horticulture greenhouse was to mist the seedlings growing in the water trays. I had a hundred foot long hose with a special misting attachment. I also sat in on any classes given by Ryan when he brought 8-10 students over from the camp to learn the mixing of minerals needed in the tray or bucket "bathes" the seedlings were placed into. We took seedlings grown in regular potting soil, cleaned the soil off the roots when there were just two inches tall and placed these naked seedling into cups that were then placed into the bath trays or the buckets for larger plants. In my spare time I read a textbook I found in the green house on general hydroponic principles and practices. I was surprised to learn that hydroponics has been expansive enterprise especially in countries like the Mideast. When Saudi Arabia for example, a predominantly desert landscape came into big oil revenues in the 1950s, their princes purchased miles of greenhouses from European and American manufacturers. They then began growing luscious food crops for their kitchens and spectacular landscaping plants and flowers for their new buildings.

When the weather turned cool in October we took most of the plants in the outside soil beds and put them either in the inside soil greenhouse or the hydroponic greenhouse.

Once Wilhelm learned I was a vegan he made sure every day that I had lettuce, tomatoes, squash and even eggplant. I really liked this guy and played pickle ball with him as often as I could. He called me Pickle Rick because he liked the name and Ryan and the rest called me Garlic Rick. I often said to him, "I work at the Will of the Wilhelm".

Before he entered the camp early this year his wife became pregnant with her first child. It was a kind of miracle conception since doctors had told her from early on that she would never be able to conceive. His case manager at first said he would be able to get out in time for the birth as he had earned some First Step Act "Good Time" credit. Apparently the warden couldn't be bothered to grant this important request. He also wouldn't allow a furlough for the birth. Wilhelm never did get to see his newborn baby boy come into this world. We were all crestfallen. In December if I'm not mistaken, Wilhelm was released to be with his family. I know you've been cheated my friend but I'm so glad you're finally home.

Chapter 13

Music

I have only one hobby, something I have been doing since middle school. I play guitar, keyboards and sing in rock and roll bands. I played gigs throughout high school at school dances and private parties. When I went off to college, I was so busy with academics and my new family that I had to stop playing in bands. I did keep playing the piano and guitar, sometimes for friends, occasionally at coffee shops for tips or fundraisers. When I reached medical school I bought a piano and have had the same bright sounding, durable Wurlitzer spinet ever since. I am better on the keyboard than the guitar but I think my forte is singing. When all four kids left home fifteen years ago, I started playing in bands again. Over the last four years, my band, Cool Jam and the Marmalades have been performing in and around Clallam County. In 2019, we played over twenty gigs at private parties, festivals, the Elks Club, the Eagles Club and that was our first year. When Covid-19 began in 2020, 'The Day the Music Died', we created our own live music events. Beginning in May, we performed outside in a parking lot on the main street in Sequim for passersby, hungry for live music so much so that every time we played we took in $200-$300 in tips. Remember these were not advertised events. We got the permission and the support of the owner of the strip mall to play. We showed up, set up, and people drove by and drove in. It was special to watch people ordered to stay home, mask up and wait nervously for the opportunity to take or ignore the vaccine, to take a break from all that stress and dance to the music.

So, to play music to an audience at Camp Sheridan, I had really only one choice at the time and that was to join one of two Chapel Bands. Due to Covid, they had closed down the "Music Room" where groups could work on their non-church band music.

The first band I learned about played on Fridays after dinner. They were very good and were on the billet as the "Power Band". They played music from Creed, good stuff; the lead singer had a powerful voice. The Chapel was a large hexagonal shaped building made of painted cinder blocks. Amplified electric bass, guitar and keyboard instruments were easily capable of excessive volume in such a place. The Power Band was no exception. As I get older, my hearing has done the opposite of what usually happens, it's gotten more sensitive so I decided to check out the other band. I checked out the Sunday "Protestant Band" run by a self-described gypsy we'll call Raphael. Raphael could play flamenco guitar and sing in that style like nobody's business. He was a gentle, positive, upbeat, middle aged soccer player who only needed a little help with his English to make the service a hit. To control our volume our bass player kept his volume down and the drummer played at the same volume. This allowed Raphael and me to keep our electric guitars at a lower volume. If you can achieve this kind of platform in a room that is essentially a large speaker box, you won't blow the audience away. We played music the congregation was used to, typical Protestant Christian songs like "This Little Light of Mine" and I sang harmony to Raphael's lead. Our drummer, Pablo spoke very little but played with a controlled perfect metronome style and added blistering quiet riffs that always made me smile. The bass player was a charming old Hawaiian I'll call Uncle who was the spiritual leader of the band. He got the audience in the right mood for each song. I played every Sunday until two weeks before I left, after the band found a replacement for me. In a sort of nostalgic way, I was a bit sad to leave these wonderful guys.

Chapter 14

My Educational Requirement

I had to register for two classes to satisfy my release requirements. I registered for an exercise class that never materialized. Regardless, just my registration satisfied one of my class requirements. I did take a "Brain Health" class which consisted of five films on various subjects relating to aspects of how the brain functions, how sleep or the lack of it affects it, how exercise affects it and such. The last film was of the most interest to me because it was about how diet affects health, not specifically of the brain, but the entire body. The film was about an Australian, Joe Cross, a CEO of a very successful corporation who did a fair amount of business in America. He had gained about eighty pounds by the time he was in his mid-forties, had high blood pressure and was on steroids for an autoimmune skin condition that threatened his life. He contacted a favorite colleague of mine Joel Fuhrman M.D. I met Joel at one of his talks sponsored by the Vegan Society of

Port Townsend, Washington only forty minutes from my clinic. Joel is a vegan physician who teaches and writes about juice and water fasting. During the first consultation and throughout the movie at subsequent consults we watched the physical transformation of Joe Cross while he drove across America on a 100-day juice fast. During this time, he lost 80 pounds and through Dr. Fuhrman's guidance was carefully weaned off steroids. [18]

I have been advocating both juice and water fasting for all thirty-six years of my career. The changes people can make from getting off blood pressure drugs to healing autoimmune diseases is very encouraging and rewarding for both the patient and the physician. This kind of healing is true naturopathic medicine.

18
https://www.imdb.com/title/tt1227378/?ref_=nm_knf_t_1

Chapter 15

My Educational Volunteering

In July, I had met another naturopathic physician Dr. Boswell, and at Ryan's suggestion we agreed to offer health classes on Saturday mornings. Boswell had an amazing collection of research on the dangerous health effects of PUFAs, polyunsaturated fatty acids on the biochemistry of the human body. He also presented scientific evidence for the negative effects of electric fields and electromagnetic fields on health. My favorite talk of his was on the harmful effect of excessive iron that accumulates in a blood protein called ferritin. In the United States, our government forces food manufacturers to add iron to all white flour and white rice foods. This process is called fortification. Most European countries forbid this practice, as they know that excess iron oxidizes (damages) tissues and the blood itself. If a person eats a normal carnivorous diet, they will get more iron than they need because of the iron in the blood of the animals eaten. Even a vegan diet provides enough iron such that the vegan does not need to store iron at all. Vegans keep their iron as serum iron ready to produce hemoglobin to carry oxygen. Storing iron as serum iron is safe, storing iron as ferritin is a ticking time bomb. It is simply crazy to add iron to the diet of 320 million meat eaters who due to eating iron rich meat get a whopping dose of iron several times a day.

Boswell and I decided to alternate our subject matter and after a month an alternative M.D. named Ronald showed up in my wing and he agreed to offer classes with us on ozone therapy, his specialty. I learned quite a bit about the benefits of ozone therapy, a practice Ronald had quite some expertise on for over twenty-five years. He used it for arthritis and infections and spoke about its benefits to the human immune system.

Each class was an hour with time for questions. My first class was on "Garlic and Larch Tree Starch" and how they can work so effectively against infections. I spoke about diabetes, arthritis, immune support and hormone disorders like hypothyroidism and adrenal exhaustion. One of my best-attended talks was about digestion and proper diet. Speaking about diet, I am sure by now you are wondering how I got along as a vegan.

Chapter 16

Chez Sheridan, the only restaurant in town

Breakfast every single day was oatios or wheat flakes with skim milk and a piece of white cake, served from 6 am to 6:20 am, as though they knew most campers would not get up for such a sugary breakfast which they didn't. I usually skipped breakfast and hoped for better fare at lunch and dinner.

The first day I came to the cafeteria for lunch I told the line, a row of five campers serving us food, that I was a vegan. The paperwork I filled out had a section for me to enter a special diet, which I did and half-heartedly expected to get something reasonable to eat. The first inmate server on the line looked at me as if I had told him I was from the planet Vega in another solar system. The second pointed to an officer standing by the door to the back of the kitchen so I went over to him and explained that I did not eat beef, pork, lamb, fish, poultry, dairy or eggs. He looked at me with a quizzical expression but had the restraint not to laugh. He simply beckoned me to follow him as he walked back to a closet, opened it and took out a vat of peanut butter. Then he smiled somewhat guiltily and said, "I'm sorry, we don't have any other vegans here that I'm aware of so we'll have to find you some plant protein. Are you willing to eat this for now?" I said OK and he had a server put some white rice, a white bun and peanut butter on a tray.

Dinner was more peanut butter with canned peas and a bun. Things were looking up, oh boy!

The next day when I came up to the first line server I got an education. "Vegan please." I asked again. "Listen guy, vegan we don't know, just say 'No Flesh', and we'll keep the meat etc. out of your tray, easier that way, OK?" Sure, I said, "No Flesh, please". Eventually, there were things I could eat, not the way Rose would make them of course, not organic, but I was in prison, complaining would do no good and when you've been working hard in horticulture all day and you've built up an appetite you eat any starch or vegetables they're willing to give you and smile about it.

Somebody in the kitchen started to take me seriously about two weeks later. By dinnertime that particular day, I was rather ravenous when I got to the line. They gave me a large helping of spicy lentil, carrot and onion stew and I almost tripped on the way to my table from surprise. It was quite good so I went back for seconds since I knew they had made it just for me. Tortillas and beans were always welcome and occasionally they served me three bean salads. Canned corn and canned carrots were common. My favorites were the baked potatoes, no fixings, just well cooked, chewy potatoes, and a nice diversion from the canned veggies. There was very little sugar at lunch and dinner, only the rare cookie or cake. I avoided the white rice and the white flour baked goods. I allowed myself spaghetti and red sauce which was served every two weeks. Once I learned how to get a reasonable amount of protein, fat and veggies from Chez Sheridan, I noticed other campers began to get curious about my selections. They would sit down at my table and ask me questions on why I ate this way. After two more weeks I started hearing "No Flesh Please" and eventually I counted about seven to eight others who had either come out of the closet or decided eating less meat was a good idea. When people at the camp would talk to me about the vegan diet, they would bring certain reasons for eating the normal food available. The most common one was, "I'm here for so many months or years, I can always eat vegan or at least vegetarian when I get out". My answer to that was, "Why eat Group One and Group Two carcinogens, acid forming, and vitality robbing animal food while you're here at all? Instead you could be eating non-carcinogenic, non-inflammation causing plant based foods since they're obviously now willing to serve them to you?" It's sort of a red pill versus blue pill question. Poison or nourishment, you choose.

Another reason was, "My wife does the cooking and she feeds me mostly vegan at home. Here it's too much work and I don't want to have to even think about it." My answer to that was, "OK, you only eat vegan because your wife is smarter than you and knows both what to feed you to keep you healthy and why the food she feeds you is healthy. Consider making decisions for yourself about your health. You are the one who is eating the excess acidic, life shortening excessive protein and fat just because you are here and she is not. If she were in a women's prison, she wouldn't make the excuse you're making."

I mentioned earlier that when I started my job in horticulture I drove around with George watering plants. George told me early on that he had arthritis. Since we lived in the same small cube together, we talked a lot and he eventually became interested in trying the vegan diet with me. I invited him to dine with me at Chez Sheridan one evening so I could help him see how to order vegan food and coach him on what to avoid, even if it was vegan, such as peanut butter. The only problem was his race. The BOP did not have any rules about what tables campers were allowed to sit in by race but the inmates created a racial separation there like the TV rooms. There were "Race Captains" so to speak in the camp. These guys were self-proclaimed inmate decision makers on all things racial. They made decisions about what sections were for white, black, Asian, Hispanic, and Islander campers. They decided which television room was for which race.

I personally thought this was *merda*, the Italian word my grandfather used instead of the American term sh** and I told George so. I told him I was going to sit at a table I had located that was in between the blacks, Hispanics, Asian/Islanders and the whites. I asked him to sit there with me as if we were regular, friendly Americans of different races regardless of the race captains if he agreed. George was my age and a retired big equipment operator. After almost seventy years, he was tired of the *merda* and happily agreed to eat with me at what we dubbed the "Multicultural" table.

The first night we ate there together, one of the white captains, there was at least three or four I found out later, came up to me and said, "Rick, you're new around here. You should not be eating here with a black man; stay within your own "car." Car I learned later is inmate slang for race. I said nothing. The next time we ate there a Hispanic camper told us this was part of the Hispanic section and we should move. We stayed put. The third time we ate there nobody said anything. After a while, we were ignored. Better yet, other people from other races came and ate with us from time to time. I don't think I could have gotten away with that in a medium facility, the racial hatred there is just too intense from what I've heard but I was pretty confident I could just wait these campers out and it worked.

A later chapter will show that, eventually a month before I was released to the halfway house Rose was able to visit me a couple times a week apart. She got the idea from her first visit to bring a vegan cookbook to the second visit. She gave it to the guard who promised to give it to the kitchen officer. She hoped that maybe the inmate kitchen staff would show some effort at making us "No Flesh" campers something with a little more variety to it.

Low and behold, within just three or four days, we started getting tofu dishes. Sautéed tofu and tofu vegetable stir-fry. It was amazing! We could not believe it and were very, very happy. I will never forget the first time it happened. My close vegetarian friend Dr. Ronald left his table and walked over to me as I was in the line about to be served. He said, "Rick you've gotta try this tofu stuff, it's fantastic, we just have to take some back to the wing in case it never happens again!"

You have to understand readers; food is a big deal in prison, especially when you cannot get what you are used to. Sure, carnivores always get what they are used to but vegetarians and vegans not so much. Until the day I was released to the halfway house, the menu for all us veggie lovers was much better. Rose had made our life less boring and more nourishing and the camp will never be the same again because of her wing and a prayer.

Chapter 17

Case Managers and Counselors

It was a common complaint by inmates that the BOP is run by for-profit contractors who save money by not hiring enough officers to handle the job properly. For example, by the time I left there were 340 inmates at the camp and only four case managers, each with a load of about eight-five campers. My case manager was almost impossible to find. He had an office but he never posted his hours or had his name on his door. I only saw him three times in four months for about five minutes each and he seemed as if he wanted me out of the office before I even arrived. He spoke very fast, explaining things as though he did not understand them himself, not answering direct questions and telling me before I could question him further that our time was over. His knowledge of the First Step Act was vague and slim, so even if you were able to ask him a question about it, he hemmed and hawed and then changed the subject.

The "counselor" was even worse, and there was only one counselor for every 180 campers. He had only three things to do: 1) get you a bunk to sleep in; 2) get you a job to work if you wanted one and were cleared by medical to have one; 3) approve of paperwork submitted by your family or friends for visitation. I was lucky to be cleared by medical staff on my third day there. I had heard of people who didn't get a visit by the medical staff for an entire month, but the census then was low (240) so they obviously had time for me. To get a job, you had to apply with an inmate such as Ryan. Ryan accepted my application and got it approved by the officer in charge of horticulture in the very first week I was there. I was given a paper with both Ryan and the officer's signature. Ryan told me to give the document to my counselor or his boss. I found out when my counselor had office hours, Sunday afternoon through Wednesday afternoon for a total of sixteen hours. Therefore, I went to his office every day during his office hours. He never showed up once. At this point, I went to his boss who promised to turn my work request into my counselor.

Ryan said I was for all intents and purposes hired since the officer had signed the document but that ultimately my counselor had to put it in the computer so I could get paid and my case manager could check it off as a task completed by me toward my release. If you work, you are out on your job for as many hours as you are needed. You are not required to be in your cube when they come by for the noon census. After some weeks went by after coming back for the 4 pm count that all workers and non-workers had to be in their cube for, two guys in my cube told me the noon officer who took the census had been asking them where I was. The inmates knew I was working in horticulture so they told the officer where I was. The census officer didn't seem to have a problem taking the other inmate's word for it that I was working and later I found out why. On the other hand, I wondered why this was happening since my counselor's boss, the second in line from the warden, had given my counselor the paperwork, which proved I was working.

After three months, I managed to see the counselor walking to his office. I only had his description and some comments as to his elusive and slacker behavior from almost everyone. Surprised, I waited a moment and knocked on his door. He ushered me in and asked me what I wanted. I told him I was working in horticulture and that his boss had sent him my document to him proving such but the noon census officers had no record of my job. Without even attempting to look for the document his boss had sent in a stack of papers on his desk he clicked on his computer and said, "So when did you start?" I explained that I had been working there for almost three months. He then entered my name in his computer saying, "Ok, as of tomorrow you're working in horticulture. Have a nice day. You can leave now". After that, the campers in my cube stopped having to stick up for me as I had officially satisfied my work requirement on their computer. The worst of this was that I was only paid for the very last of my four months at the camp. Hey, if you were paid **$5.26 for a month's work**, the loss of three months' wages would stick in your craw don't you think? Sometimes I wonder if I had not accidentally seen this guy sneaking into his office if I'd have ever gotten out of prison.

Chapter 18

Visitation

After Rose sent my counselor properly filled out requests for visitation three separate times that took over three months, I finally got an email from him that I would be able to see my wife. It's funny; I was emailing Rose almost every day so when Saturday rolled around and she came to the visitation room, I figured we wouldn't have anything to say to each other. Visitors were allowed to come as early as 9 am and leave by 3 pm. The visitation room is a large room across the hall from the administration and medical offices. It doubles as a space during the week for the classes for illegal drug salesmen or drug addicts. All sorts of posters are on the walls promoting positive living ideas for the inmate students. One-half of the camp's population is in this program or trying to get into it. If they successfully complete the class work over a nine-month period, they get one whole year off their sentence.

To get ready for the event, my friends gave me the protocol weeks in advance. You find your best pants and shirt and you press them as best you can. Since they don't let you use an iron, I put them on an empty top bunk bed weighed down by pounds of legal documents I had received from my attorneys. You use your best shoes and if you don't have nice shoes, you borrow a pair from a friend. You wash twice the night before and use deodorant. I did everything exactly as outlined, including borrowing shoes from a friend. I have never been away from Rose that long and I wanted to spruce up as best I could.

The drive down from Port Angeles to Camp Sheridan is about five hours so Rose stayed at a family member's house in northern Oregon Friday night. She then drove an hour and came into the room at about 10 am. During visitation, the visitors go in the front door and the inmates go in through a side door hallway. The officer has you take anything you might have in your pockets out, any jewelry, scarf, anything.

The visitation room has four sections on each long wall so that eight total inmates and their visitors can meet. Each section has two chairs facing each other and a short square table between the chairs. You are allowed a brief hug and short kiss and then you need to stay seated until you're ready to leave. We talked and laughed together from about 10 am to 3 pm when we all had to leave. During this five-hour period, inmates that I knew were positioned on either side of us. Their partners brought toddlers with them who were quite entertaining as they crawled around, keeping the couples rather busy but loving every minute. It was a very special time for Rose and I, you know how they say, "Parting makes the heart grow fonder". We were both surprised we stayed there so long and glad at the same time. A week later, we did it all over again and two weeks later, I left for the halfway house.

Chapter 19

Getting Out of Prison into a Different Kind of Prison

On October 29, I was called into an office to see a case manager I had never heard of nor had anyone else. At about 3pm on a Thursday, I heard over the intercom, "Inmate Richard Marschall, prison number such and such, report to building five, wing five." I went up to this office and a new face told me to sit down and that I was going to be released to a halfway house in Tacoma, a city an hour south of Seattle in four days, November 7th to be exact. He said I would need to wake up at 3 am and be driven to Portland, Oregon, by the camp inmate driver. From there, I would take a Greyhound bus to Tacoma and a taxi to the halfway house. He showed me a copy of a purchased bus ticket. He explained that I would be given a prison issued VISA card with money from my prison account used to spend on commissary items. He explained that I would be given fourteen dollars cash for the taxi fare. He said all this in less than five minutes, had me sign something and ushered me out the door, no time for questions, typical.

I was expecting early release to home confinement by December 6, according to the computed data sheet. Home confinement in Washington means they have you install an app on your phone and you must stay at your home unless you request a pass. Passes were routinely allowed for shopping, work or other functions approved by a probation officer at the halfway house. The wardens are required by the First Step Act to release inmates this way unless they had broken any of the rules and regulations during my time there. If that had happened in my case, my case manager would have informed me of such. Nothing like that happened because I followed the rules, met my work and education requirements and was well over sixty years old.

Regardless of the warden sending me to the halfway house, I was still happy just to be getting out to anywhere. I was in shock but smiling and crying at the same time. I do that when I get emotional, it's not very manly I guess but that's just who I am at seventy-one years old. Rose says it has something to do with my astrological sign being Cancer. Whether it's true or not, it is what it is.

As I walked around the campus, I met friends and told them the news. They were happy for anyone, leaving, including me, leaving, even if their date was delayed. This was always a time for smiles and pats on the back from even campers you barely knew, and news travels fast.

The next day, I sat in Chez Sheridan with some friends and I realized I was getting out of an actual prison to somewhere else, an entire month early. Had the warden cared to do his job, the law said I needed to stay in the camp for five months and eleven days, which is exactly two thirds of my eight-month sentence. If in fact this occurred, I would be out to a Halfway house in four months and eleven days. Why was this happening? No one, not even Ryan understood why they wanted to release me to a halfway house an entire month early; I was still being given more freedom sooner than expected. Remember this is regardless of the fact that I'm still NOT getting any Congressional First Step credit for being an old guy, the two months the U.S. government expected the prison wardens to follow. No, warden would rather go along with the federal judge and keep me under some kinds of federal detention for the full 8 months.

As November 7 came closer, I decided to throw myself a sort of going away party. I let people know that I would be in my cube Sunday evening around 8 pm, the night before I would be leaving at 3 am Monday morning. I laid out a spread of treats, chips, hummus and salsa on the 3-foot-high locker top closest to the hallway between the cubes. Over the next two hours' friends dropped in to eat and share some memories, as well as give me some hugs and pats on the back. There was a lot of, "we're gonna miss you Garlic Rick but don't ever come back here" kind of thing. There was also some exchanging of contacts for well into the future when we're all out and its "safe" to contact each other.

I had a very special relationship with Ronald, the alternative medical doctor whom I was lucky enough to get to know over the last month. We were spiritually connected, both vegetarians, and shared very similar physician skills and experiences. We liked to play pickle ball and walk the track together. He agreed to stay up late with me for a while and play Scrabble to help me stay awake. He's very good at Scrabble and unfortunately, I lost more often than I won. At about 2 pm we were done so I told him to hit the sack. I knew I was too excited as most inmates are on the day they leave prison; I couldn't sleep anyway.

I was sitting on the toilet at 2:50 am when someone started banging on the door of my stall. "Hey Marschall, it's time for you to leave, you don't get to stay here anymore". I hadn't met this officer before but those were possibly the sweetest words I've ever heard since I arrived there. I had a sack of books and a sack of personal items with me so I hurriedly followed him 200 feet from the front door of the Camp to the Detention Center, the place I had originally had surrendered to. I was given an envelope with fourteen dollars, a debit card with sixty-four dollars and a Greyhound bus ticket.

I got in the van with one other inmate who was on his way north to Portland then south to a Eugene Oregon halfway house there, even though he lived two hours east of Seattle! His bus would be leaving Portland at 7 am, hence the 3 am departure from Sheridan. As the inmate driver rolled on to Portland, I learned they had given him only four dollars in cash for his taxi from the Eugene Greyhound station to the halfway house. I asked him how much he had on the prison debit card they gave him and he said only three dollars. Before you leave a federal prison they transfer any money you had in your prison "bank account" into a special prison debit card. I couldn't leave this poor guy without a viable way to get from Eugene to the halfway house so I just gave him my fourteen dollars cash, figuring I'd get some cash when I got to Portland on my debit card since there was plenty of money on the card.

Sheridan is a little over an hour from Portland so we got into the downtown area at about 4:30 am. When we arrived in Portland, the driver let us out at the Amtrak train station. We asked the driver where the Greyhound bus station was and he said he didn't really know and suggested we ask someone at the train station. We walked into the train station and a security guard said he didn't know either. This is November in the Northwest, and it was cold outside, in the mid thirties. We asked him if we could stay inside until the ticket counter opened up to ask a clerk. He apologized and told us we had to leave, Portland, the friendly Northwest city. At 4:40 am, we have no choice but to be out in the cold, dark deserted downtown Portland back streets. Then it starts to rain.

This all happened so fast that Rose had not had time to get me any warm clothing through the mail. I had two sweatshirts and a pair of pants. We walked around downtown Portland looking for shelter with little luck and later a bathroom with no luck. There wasn't even an early open coffee shop or public restroom nearby. I knew where the downtown Willamette River park was from our location and that there was a public bathroom there. So we headed there praying hard it would be open, getting soaked from a heavy rain and cold wind. We walked/ran two miles and lucked out. After relieving ourselves we walked back another two miles, and by now its 6:00 am.

We found an open coffee shop to try to dry out. I bought him some coffee and a pastry on my prison debit card and, forty minutes later, he left for his 7 am bus ride. I'm not scheduled to leave Portland for Tacoma until 11 am so I have to find something to do for four hours. The rain stopped and I figured I need to get some cash to pay the taxi driver in Tacoma for a ride to my halfway house. So I headed out to find a bank with an automatic teller machine. I found plenty of closed banks with outside ATMs but not one that would honor this new prison debit card! Now I'm in a pickle, I have a Greyhound ticket to Tacoma but nothing for the taxi.

I went to a Safeway grocery store and tried buying something there and getting cash back. The same response, although the coffee shop took my card neither the Safeway nor the bank ATMs would. I'm confused and a bit stressed at this point so I told my story to the cashier, and she was kind enough to let me use the store phone at customer service. I called the number on the back of the debit card and they apologized for their screw-up and fixed the problem. Right then I was able to get cash from the helpful Safeway cashier. Remember readers, I gave the cash I needed originally to the inmate I had been traveling with. What's that saying, no good deed goes unpunished? Anyway it was an adventure and I've always lived by the adage, "Stay Positive and Good Things Will Happen".

It took me three hours and miles of walking around downtown Portland to get the cash I needed. That left me with an hour to wait somewhere while it's still raining for the bus to show up on a street near the train station. I went back to the coffee shop a couple blocks from the Greyhound 'street station', ordered another drink and waited an hour reading. Then I walked down to the 'street station' to see things happening.

Two men were walking up and down the road where the buses stopped, checking passenger tickets. The bus arrived at 11:10 am and it took about three hours to reach Tacoma, Washington. After a ten-minute taxi ride to the Port of Tacoma neighborhood, I finally arrived at the halfway house.

On arrival, I spent an hour filling out countless forms as if this satellite of the Federal Bureau of Prisons had never heard of me before. I next met my case manager who confirmed that I would be there until February 10 which was only fourteen days short of my full eight-month sentence. I showed them the paper I had from the prison case manager that said I was eligible for a one-third off my sentence "elderly offender early release" option. The halfway house director said "Well, the warden has 'discretionary' power to deny early release." I countered with, "On what basis can he deny it? I was a model prisoner, broke no rules, worked a job as required, took the classes requested. How can he possibly deny me this 2018 Congressionally authorized option? "As I said, replied the half-way house official, 'discretionary

power'. Even my attorneys had no luck making any sense of this by attempting to contact the warden who never responded, nor the Federal Bureau of Prison center in Texas who did respond with 'discretionary power'. I'm pretty sure 'discretionary power' in the Federal Bureau of Prison system in my case could be easily translated to mean: "the warden was to overworked or lazy or both to properly do his job respecting my constitutional 'right to freedom from unlawful detention' ".

Chapter 20

Life in the Halfway House

A halfway house is very different from a prison. First, you can have a cell phone. Second, you can have a laptop. This is a big deal because in the camp no inmate had access to the internet through a computer. Computers in the classroom or the library were only available for writing documents or emailing your vetted list of contacts. Third, you can leave the place for up to eight hours a day and spend forty-eight hours each week with your family and friends. For some of the twenty men at this facility it was possible and easy. Unfortunately, only three of us had cars so the rest had to take a bus or get a ride by family or friends. The bus stop was a good walk away so not a lot of takers there, especially in the winter.

The reason in my opinion might be that most half-way house residents didn't have cars parallels with the white-collar/drug dealer/user ration of 15-85 I observed at the camp. Most white collar inmates at the camp had money and vehicles to come home to. Most drug dealers had lost their money in the federal government stings that resulted in their incarceration.

Half-way house residents are encouraged to find local jobs. Residents are **not** allowed to work their own businesses. Before I went in the BOP system, I had had a successful 32 year licensed physician practice and next a successful 4 year Health Coach business taken away from me in the camp and through to the halfway house. My half-way house counselor advised me to apply for a job and gave me a list of local possibilities. I was curious if getting a job was a negotiable consideration or an actual federal prison system requirement. Good News, it was negotiable. I explained that at the time of my original incarceration my wife Rose had been able to kept my existing clients (patients) supplied with plant-based medicines as usual and that I had savings at home and would be getting my social security back when left the federal prison system in a few months. The response was, OK! He then asked me what I would be doing with my time while I was there since I had a car and was allowed to leave for 8 hours a day. I explain what I decided to do next but my counselor then gave me the tour which ended showing me my room. It was another cinder block construction but with high ceilings with windows so high you could only see treetops, tower tops and a second story business. There were four beds, four lockers, but only one roommate.

I am seventy-one years old, I've been in a prison camp for the last four months sleeping on a dead, lumpy thin mattress. Now I'm in a halfway house sleeping again on a hard thicker bed that is forty feet from a 5G cell tower. Believe it or not, the prison camp bed was more comfortable and there weren't any cell towers nearby cooking me in invisible electromagnetic pro-inflammatory wave forms.

So now for the first time since I can remember I'm waking up with back pain and not allowed to do what I do best, 'Health Coaching'. So, I started going to the gym and writing this book. If I couldn't provide health care yet to needy people I could at least expose the corruption, greed and mean spiritedness of the establishment.

To relieve the 'hard bed back pain' I woke up every morning and went the YMCA in downtown Tacoma. It was only a 12 minute drive to a very modern and well endowed facility. Boy, to drive again! How fun!! During the first two weeks there I also took long drives along the Tacoma waterfront just to feel the steering wheel and the accelerator again.

I started with floor exercises in the "Toning Room" for thirty minutes. Then I begin walking for an hour on the quarter mile track above the indoor basketball court. This helped my low back pain from the nasty bed to become sixty percent improved. After six minutes in the steam room, I am almost back to normal and on to the library.

The nicest library I found wasn't in Tacoma; it was in a community next door called University Place. I didn't understand why they called it that, since in my travels around the city, I never saw a university anywhere and they're generally pretty hard to miss. I looked it up in Wikipedia and found that in the 1800s, the University of Puget Sound purchased land there to build a campus but ended up selling it back to Tacoma for $11,000. University Place remained unincorporated until the City Of University Place was formed in 1995 and now has a population of 35,000. I like this area, it's on the water with the Puget Sound on the West side and the city of Tacoma on the north and east side.

The University Place library is two hundred feet from a Whole Foods, which is convenient for a vegan who gets very little safe and nourishing food from the halfway house. After a month of eating only the vegetables, pasta and white bread they had available, one of the staff observed me avoiding the meat and said, "Are you a vegetarian?" I said, "Yes, I filled that information out on the litany of forms you guys gave me when I first arrived". "Oh, he replied, I'm sorry we missed that. Well we'll get you a special diet from now on."

Ever since then, they have been giving me three plastic containers with class-one-carcinogen fake meats, (made with isolated soy protein), some vegetables and an apple or orange. I told them I would not eat the fake meat but they said they did not think they could do anything about that. I was going to give them some information about how to feed a vegan properly but after talking with the staff I learned that by the time they could get around to providing me healthier choices I'd be home.

Regardless, I've been supplementing with organic oatmeal, organic multi-grain bread, and occasional raids on the Whole Foods hot food/salad bar.

There are some beautiful parts of Tacoma. When the sun is out and there is little wind, instead of walking the YMCA track indoors I drove out to Point Ruston or Point Defiance to walk in the fresh sea air. The drive there takes you along the south side of the Port of Tacoma waterway, which has many parks overlooking the beachfront. As you drive west, you can see trains, boats, and joggers to your right as you look across to the north shore of the port. When you return the train tracks are up on a short bluff to your right. Along the south shore there are many large, fine seafood restaurants built on old piers with names like "Harbor Lights," "Stanley and Seafort" and "Shenanigans." Just before you reach Point Defiance, you see large high-rise condominiums at Point Ruston, a modern community with its own grocery, restaurants, ice cream parlor, cinema and large paved waterfront walkway out to the ferry landing. The ferry goes over to Vashon Island, a cozy little island community for the rich retirees, co-housing commuters and other well-to-do islanders.

Point Defiance is a very large recreation area that contains a long mostly paved waterfront trail, a restaurant on the water, and an angler's bait and tackles shop. You can walk due west until the land ends and see the marinas of Gig Harbor that span across a channel of the Puget Sound that flows under the Tacoma Narrows Bridge. These walks in the brisk winter air are my best memories of my stay at this halfway house.

Chapter 21

Barley

When I arrived at the halfway house, I found an inmate there I knew from Camp Sheridan who had arrived about twelve weeks before I did. His name shall be Barley and he is about 60 years old. He's a short fellow but a hard worker. He has an injury to his back that caused his spinal column to solidify such that instead of standing vertical he bends forward from the mid back at about a 45-degree angle. Regardless, shortly after he arrived there, he got a job in a warehouse picking stuff up and moving it to somewhere else. He walks to the bus to get to work and on days he doesn't work, he walks around Tacoma. I marvel at this man's stamina and work ethic.

When I was in the camp I watched Barley walk the quarter mile track for at least an hour a day. Inmates there told me that Barley could do a **double** back flip off any of the wooden park benches on the campus. I thought to myself when I heard this, boy I have gotta see that! Barley would walk the camp track a lot so one day, after walking with him for several miles I asked him if he would show me how he did it. He agreed and when he was ready, we left the track and walked over to the nearest camp park bench. He explained to me that he first did this when he saw a correction officer walking by that he didn't particularly like. He told me I needed to pretend that I was the cop because that would stimulate the energy he needed to perform the feat. I said fine, so I stared intently at him with a gnarly face. After he saw my grimace, he stood up on the bench, facing away from me; he bent down on his knees in a deep crouch as if he were ready to jump high in the air. Then he managed to raise both arms behind his back and he flipped me the bird from each hand.

Ok, I said to myself, **double** (2 handed) while your **back** is turned to someone, flipping the **bird**…the infamous Barley **double backflip**!

I could not stop laughing! I got punked, but when he told me the name of the officer he did it too, well, I understood why he did it. This joke was for newbies and quite a well preserved camp tradition apparently because at least nine people had passed this stunt along to me keeping a straight face, never letting on that I was being duped.

Well, here he was, and as the weeks went by, we rekindled what originally was an unrequited friendship. Barley is a friendly and cheerful fellow with a good word to say. I wish him the very best.

Chapter 22

Frank

One week ago, as I was coming back from the library, I found an inmate I've named Frank sitting in the dayroom. Frank is a Cameroon-American who was there in my wing when I arrived in early July. Frank is the nicest guy, easy to talk to and very friendly. When we were at the camp, after he learned that I could play a medley of 'La Bamba' and 'Twist and Shout', he organized the wing to sing along with us on Saturday nights. It was a highlight of the week for my wing, smiles everywhere; even if you didn't join in singing it helped make the 30 of us feel like we were at a party at home for a few minutes.

Frank worked in the kitchen and was given a 'shot' by his case manager for taking some food from the cafeteria, something everyone did. When you receive a shot for breaking the rules, you get a short hearing with your case officer and another officer present. I helped him strategize for his hearing and after that support, we became fast friends. Yesterday he told me Camp Sheridan let twelve inmates out all at once to home confinement, the very thing I was supposed to get on December 6. Better yet, they were going to let him out to home confinement the next day!

Frank just left today, and before his girlfriend picked him up, we shook hands, hugged and I wished him the very best. But it's mid-January and I'm still here with a month to go.

Chapter 23

Getting out to Freedom

I am very close now, only ten days to go. I'm on "countdown" where people around me, including the halfway house staff are greeting me with, "You're almost out here, aren't you?" It's a nice thing to hear.

I've been building a list of things I need to do first when I'm released:

1. See my chiropractor. The BOP doesn't let you use your own health insurance or Medicare to get the healthcare you need. They have their own health insurance. The BOP doctor who cleared me for work backs at the camp told me as he led me to his office, "You should accept that the BOP has the very worst health plan currently available in the United States." That was so nice to hear during my first official week in the camp. Prison healthcare certainly doesn't cover chiropractors or naturopathic physicians at their prisons or halfway houses. Cruel and unusual punishment? Should inmates at a federal prison camp be denied the same health and medical services available to un-incarcerated Americans? I'm not talking about massage therapy but question is, "why does the government restrict health and medical services to medical doctors over chiropractors, naturopathic physicians and

acupuncturists?" These alternative practitioners are covered by most insurance plans and in many states. Chiropractic is covered by Medicare in all 50 states. I will go back to seeing my chiropractor twice a month when I get out because that care has helped keep me from needing a need or shoulder replacement over the last 6 years.

2. See my physical therapist, also not covered by the federal prison system. Again, care that has helped me to prevent major surgeries. I'll just need a few sessions with him to get me back on track as the exercises he teaches I've been doing and will continue to do.
3. Restart my Health Coach practice. I have existing patients that will have been waiting 8 months to consult with me. They've relied on my wife Rose to continue receiving their natural plant based medicines and food supplements but some require periodic

health coaching and all require occasional adjustments to their health plans.
4. Take Rose out to dinner for Valentine's Day. I'll be getting out almost right on Valentine's Day so this will be a super time to rekindle our 44th year of marriage.
5. Publish this book.
6. Ride the Chilly Hilly bicycle ride on Bainbridge Island at the end of February.
7. Play pickle ball in the indoor courts in Port Angeles and Sequim.

Chapter 24

Other Early Treatment physicians

A list of the doctors around the country who were branded as 'mis-informationists', forced to remove their lifesaving information online, had their license threatened by their medical board, had their board certifications removed, had their license removed or even were sent to jail, can be viewed below:

- Simone Gold M.D. J.D. Founder Simone Gold, MD, JD, FABEM, is a board-certified emergency physician who has worked on the front lines of the coronavirus pandemic. She is the author of the provocative, top-selling book *I Do Not Consent: My Fight against Medical Cancel Culture*. Gold graduated from Chicago Medical School before attending Stanford University Law School to earn her Juris Doctorate. Her advocacy revolves around inalienable rights of freedom: bodily sovereignty, voluntary informed consent, free speech. In addition, she vehemently opposes bureaucratic encroachments on the doctor-patient relationship and overzealous state pharmacy boards. Dr. Gold was sentenced to sixty days for protesting on the Capitol Hill steps on January 6, 2021, the persecution of doctors for offering early treatment of Covid and the government's actions to thwart physicians and pharmacists from treating Covid patients with repurposed medications.

- Peter McCullough M.D. professor of Medicine at Baily University School of Medicine, author of more papers on the nature of the Covid virus and the early treatment of Covid than anyone worldwide. His information was used in Congressional hearings to attempt to stop the government efforts to discourage and persecute physicians doing early Covid-19 treatment. Dr. McCullough has been under investigation by his medical board for sharing his contentious views on Covid vaccines. The only problem with this shameless journalism if one actually follows the research is, Peter McCullough M.D. shared **truthful evidence** about the vaccines. Tthere's nothing "contentious" about his views, they're simple science

based facts. Eventually Dr. McCullough's board certifications were removed. [19] [20]
- Robert Karas M.D. provided life-saving Ivermectin to inmates at a state prison in Arkansas. The Kansas Medical Board is currently investigating his actions. If you know anything about medical care available in prisons and I do, you should understand there are long waiting lines and often no treatments available. Signs tacked on the wall of the Sheridan Federal prison where I was incarcerated said, "We will not see inmates with upper respiratory colds or flues, buy over the counter medicines." Inmates had to be almost comatose to get a visit to the local hospital while I was there.

---

[19] https://link.springer.com/article/10.1007/s00392-022-02129-5

[20] https://thetexan.news/dallas-cardiologist-peter-mcculloughs-medical-certifications-revoked-by-american-board-of-internal-medicine/

Many would have really appreciated Dr. Karas's willingness to provide Ivermectin. [21]
- Sheri Tenpenny D.O. for offering early treatment for Covid-19. [22]
- Joseph Mercola D.O. was forced to take down factual but government annoying information on his website providing early treatment for Covid-19 [23]
- Edith Behr M.D., licensed physician and surgeon in Pennsylvania was fired from the Tower Health Medical Group for prescribing Ivermectin earlier this year in February 2022. [24]

[21] https://www.nwahomepage.com/news/patients-support-doctor-who-has-been-prescribing-ivermectin-to-inmates-with-covid-19/

[22] https://www.medpagetoday.com/special-reports/exclusives/101529

[23] https://www.organicconsumers.org/news/did-lockdowns-cause-increased-mortality-rates

[24] https://www.ldnews.com/story/news/2022/02/03/lebanon

- Eric Depute D.C. harassed by the FTC for offering early Covid-19 treatment. [25]
- Senator Mark Stephen M.D. was put under investigation by the Kansas State Medical board for prescribing Ivermectin in January of 2022. [26]
- John Littell M.D Florida physician who has extensive frontline clinical experience with Ivermectin was suspended from one hospital for his courageous, early treatment of Covid-19. [27]

-woman-touts-dr-edith-behr-to-prescribe-ivermectin-hydroxychloroquine/9313726002/

[25] https://www.webmd.com/lung/news/20210422/first-person-charged-under-covid-false-claims-law

[26] https://apnews.com/article/coronavirus-pandemic-health-business-worms-legislature-054e83c1a4d69704b4ed6508c301dd18

[27] https://www.wesh.com/article/florida-doctor-claims-hes-treated-3000-covid-19-patients-with-human-version-of-ivermectin/39302154

These are just a few examples of physicians across America who have braved the persecution by Big Pharma through their enforcers, the state boards of health, the Federal Trade Commission, the AMA and Big Pharma. If your state board of health finds a doctor prescribing mercury, birthday cake, or nail polish for the flu, OK, I agree, it should be investigated. However, when many studies show a treatment is safe and effective and is urgently needed to save lives well, the members on the board of health become the members of the "board of death". There's no other way to describe a group of thugs in suits or white coats that go around harassing and persecuting physicians from treating people safely by keeping them out of the hospital and alive.

Physicians have a private relationship with their patients. Doctors do not even have to share that relationship with authorities unless there is a report of malpractice, not a report that a physician encourages early treatment of a disease over being vaccinated with a new vaccine that has only an animal study behind it. How would you like it if the federal government had the authority to defrock your minister because the agency told him praying for help from a mythical person was "misinformation" or that drinking a bit of wine at a service was against health and safety policies? When government agencies can threaten or take the license to practice away from progressive, frontline physicians, you are living under an oppressive, dangerous government and your leaders are acting in a corrupt way.

The upside though is that there are states fighting this State Board of Health Gestapo-like policy. The following states have passed or have bills in their legislatures to protect the physicians in their state from persecution:

Tennessee

HB 1870/SB 1880 prevents medical licensing boards or subcommittees from taking any disciplinary action against physicians related to COVID-19 treatment, if the provider thinks the treatment is in the patient's best interest. HB 2506/SB 2621 allows doctors, PAs, and APRNs to prescribe Ivermectin, and lets pharmacists dispense it, without facing discipline from licensing boards. HB 2744/SB 2630 stipulates the same for pharmacies to dispense Ivermectin and hydroxychloroquine.

The state's medical board pulled their policy with the FSMB language from its website in response to pressure from Republican lawmakers. According to a Tennessee state representative who spoke to *MedPage Today* previously, the medical board was being given too much power, and he had heard from doctors in his area that it was "just unheard of and unprecedented that this board of medical examiners would review things that we're saying."

Virginia

HB 102/SB 711 keeps medical licensing boards from disciplining providers who prescribe FDA-approved drugs for off-label use.

Washington

HB 2065 allows providers, including naturopathic practitioners, to recommend or prescribe hydroxychloroquine, ivermectin, the steroid budesonide, monoclonal antibodies, zinc, vitamin D, and vitamin C for COVID-19 without facing disciplinary action.

West Virginia

HB 4309 lets providers prescribe hydroxychloroquine, chloroquine, or ivermectin off-label; specifies that no action can be taken against prescribers; and that such prescriptions do not constitute "unprofessional conduct or otherwise grounds for discipline. HB 4455/SB 605 allows pharmacists to prescribe ivermectin through a doctor or APRN standing order, and states that no data on the information sheet about the drug can discourage the use of ivermectin. Medical boards would not be able to take action against the standing orders.

Wisconsin

Introduction of a bill that would amend the state statute to protect healthcare providers from any action from their credentialing board in the Department of Safety and Professional Services. The bill proposes that no credentialing board can retaliate, discriminate, or otherwise take any action against a provider for expressing their "professional opinions." [28]

These states have introduced these bills due to the criminal interference created by their respective boards of health. Many other states such as Florida,

---

[28] https://www.medpagetoday.com/special-reports/exclusives/97237

Mississippi, Alabama, Georgia, Texas, and Oklahoma have governors and legislatures that **already** believe their physicians have the constitutional right to treat their patients and their boards of health have the good sense to let these physicians do their jobs.

Chapter 25

The Covid-19 Players

I am going to share the research I have done over the last three years on the origins of both the virus and the vaccine to my understanding. To unravel the Covid-19 virus development and the Covid-19 vaccine, we have to understand the history of the players that have been involved in the AIDS virus, the SARS virus (severe acute respiratory syndrome), the MERS virus (Middle East Respiratory Syndrome), and the SARS-Cov-2 virus (the Covid-19 virus). I have listed them in the historical order in which they came on the scene:

- Robert Kennedy Jr. is a pioneer in environmental law who serves as chief prosecuting attorney for the Hudson River Keeper organization and as senior attorney for the National Resources Defense Council. He is also clinical professor and supervising attorney at the Environmental Litigation Clinic at Pace University School of Law in New York. Around 2005, parents of vaccine-injured children began encountering Kennedy's speeches and writings about the toxic mercury-based preservative thimerosal. They embraced new hope that this environmental champion would finally expose the truth about vaccine injury and win justice for injured children. Kennedy is known for his fierce and relentless brand of environmental activism and his advocacy for transparent government and rigorous science. He is now applying his tenacious energies and sophisticated strategies to exposing fraud and corruption within the Centers for Disease Control and Prevention (CDC) and the pharmaceutical industry. In 2016, he launched his non-profit, Children's Health Defense, with vaccine safety advocates Lyn Redwood and Laura Bono, legends themselves among parents of vaccine-injured children. His latest book "The Real Anthony Fauci: Bill Gates, Big Pharma, and the Global War on Democracy and Public Health" provides a detailed factual paper trail of Big Government's Covid-19 disease and vaccine attack on Americans. [29]

- Dr. Judy Mikovits PhD is a research scientist at NIAID who showed the association of the XMRV virus with Chronic

---

[29] https://childrenshealthdefense.org/
https://www.amazon.com/Deluxe-Boxed-Set-Democracy-Childrens-ebook/dp/B09VQTK24G

Fatigue Syndrome. She also conducted research that exposed Anthony Fauci as the man solely responsible for the development of the bioengineered Sars-Cov-2 and the Covid-19 virus. [30]

- Frank Ruscetti PhD. is an immunologist who worked on discovering the first effective treatment for AIDs, Interleukin 2. He also worked on interferon for AIDs and encouraged its use for the early treatment of Covid-19. [31]

---

[30] https://www.google.com/search?q=judy+mikovits+books&rlz=1C1GCEA_enUS1041&oq=judy+mikovits+books&aqs=chrome..69i57j0i22i30l4.6064j0j7&sourceid=chrome&ie=UTF-8

[31] https://www.thriftbooks.com/w/ending-plague-a-scholars-obligation-in-an-age-of-corruption_kent-heckenlively_francis-w-ruscetti/26822381/item/55319164/?gclid=Cj0KCQiAlKmeBhCkARIsAHy7WVuL7ioh-MfThp10DGYl3PEJtYp4e2NRXD5l4o0_H-6gU_NF8TwC4e0aArYoEALw_wcB#idiq=55319164&edition=48673917

- Robert Malone M.D. worked at Pfizer Pharmaceuticals and is the primary scientist accredited with the development of the first mRNA vaccine. He has gone on record as saying the misuse of mRNA technology has led to countless Covid-19 vaccine deaths around the world and has made it his mission to educate the world about the dangers of the Covid-19 vaccine.
- David Martin M.D. developed one of the first cancer lasers in the world and is the CEO of MCAM, the largest of one of five underwriters of intangible assets in the world such as patents. He has followed the United States Patent Office history of Anthony Fauci's gain of function additions to the wild coronavirus. He has proof of Fauci's criminal behavior.
- Peter Kory M.D. Leader in the early treatment of Covid-19 using Ivermectin with other physicians around the world. [32]

[32] https://www.youtube.com/watch?v=k8RyV3VEDKI

- Mathew Miller Skow & Nicholas Stumphauzer, filmmakers of "Died Suddenly", November 2022. Well documented film of embalmers who have found white fibrous clots never seen before in Covid-19 vaccinated dead bodies; Whistleblowers from the armed services showing increased deaths from strokes and heart attacks of young vaccinated soldiers; More whistleblowers revealing 300-700% increased fetal deaths that began 9 months after Covid-19 vaccinations were approved for pregnant mothers. [33]
- Rand Paul M.D., senator from Kentucky, senior member of the Senate Health, Education, Labor and Pensions committee. He is a tireless investigator of Anthony Fauci.
- Roger Marshall M.D., senator from Kansas member of the Senate Health, Education,

---

[33] https://rumble.com/v1wac7i-world-premier-died-suddenly.html

Labor and Pensions committee. Proponent of early treatment for Covid-19 and investigator of Anthony Fauci.
- Robert Gallo, beginning in the 1970s worked as the top virologist at the National Cancer Institute AIDS began in 1978 in Africa and by 1982 arrived in New York City. Gallo took credit for isolation of the HIV virus isolate when in fact it was originally discovered by Luc Montagnier of the Pasteur Institute in France. He also took credit for the discovery of Interleukin 2 by Frank Ruscetti M.D., the first effective treatment for the AIDS virus. More on Frank later.
- National Health Federation, which began opposing Big Pharma in the early 60s, investigated the virus even before it was released by Wuhan due to the efforts especially of its president, Scott Tips esquire. Much of Scott's efforts are reviewed in this book.

- Jonathan Wright N.D. M.D. physician, early in the pandemic Dr. Wright was instrumental in creating a large healing center staffed with naturopathic physicians that creatively and quietly improved the immune response to the pandemic over the last 3 years.
- Ryan Cole M.D. is a private pathologist based out of Utah who, along with Robert Malone M.D. has spread the word around America of the dangers of the vaccine in general. These two tireless health warriors went on a nationwide tour speaking to parents in early 2022 about the dangers of the gene shot to their children.
- The National Institute of Health (NIH) in Bethesda Maryland is the highest governmental health research agency in the United States. It oversees the Center for Disease Control (CDC) in Atlanta Georgia, the National Institute of Allergy and Infectious Disease (NIAID) in Bethesda,

Maryland, and the National Cancer Institute (NCI) located in Bethesda.

- Anthony Fauci M.D. is the director of the National Institute of Immunology and Allergy Diseases (NIAID). Since the 1980s, Fauci has stepped over fellow researchers to secure his position as the chief of NIAID by fraudulently taking credit for the work of the great virologists/immunologists working under him like Frank Ruscetti and Judy Mikovits. Fauci stood in the way of the use of Interferon and IL-2, immune system biologics that proved effective for the treatment of Covid-19. Instead, he waited an entire year and only allowed the highly toxic Ebola virus drug Remdesivir to be approved for Covid-19 in January of 2021. He also encouraged the prosecution of physicians who used early treatments for Covid-19. He, along with the FDA created the approval in January of 2021 of the first

Covid-19 mRNA vaccine and subsequent vaccines throughout 2021 and 2022. [34]
- Ralph Baric PhD is a virologist at both the University of North Carolina at Chapel Hill and Fort Dietrich military research facility in Maryland. He was Anthony Fauci's main co-conspirator doing the actual work to weaponize the wild coronavirus.
- Bill Gates, who has built a second fortune over the last 20 years since he entered the vaccine business, has a stake in vaccines and has been around the world encouraging countries like India and sub-Saharan Africa to accept his vaccine programs. Bill boasts that he has donated 10 billion dollars from the Bill and Melinda Gates Foundation between 2010 and 2020. What he fails to tell you though is that the Bill and Melinda Trust has accumulated 40 billion dollars

---

[34] https://www.medrxiv.org/content/10.1101/2022.04.05.22273167v1.full

from sales of vaccines over that same period.
- Peter Dazak PhD, zoologist, member of the WHO team that investigated the origin of Covid-19, admitted that Fauci authorized through the National Institute of Health the money allocated for gain of function funding given to the Wuhan Virology Institute in China. [35]
- Deborah Birx M.D. was the White House Coronavirus Response Coordinator. Deborah was a major promoter of the Covid-10 mRNA vaccine.

Enter Anthony Fauci who decided in 1999 to begin bioengineering the natural coronavirus according to the United States Patent Office filings he made.

---

[35] https://www.wnd.com/2021/06/fauci-funded-scientist-chinese-colleagues-created-killer-coronavirus/

To bioengineer a virus you add pieces of other virus code to the natural genetic code of the virus you are working with. A virus is a piece of genetic code encased in a protein-fat membrane.

It is shaped like a ball and is measured in nanometers, one thousandth of the size of a living cell. The shapes sticking off the virus body are the proteins. In the case of Covid-19, they are called spike proteins and are toxic to human cells. Inside a virus is a molecule of genetic material called mRNA. Since scientists today can splice genetic material from one virus into another virus like the coronavirus, it took a foolish arrogant virologist like Fauci and other scientists from the CDC to risk the lives of everyone in the world to do just that. Fauci started with the wild or natural coronavirus from the animal world; Coronaviruses up until this point were only causing disease in dogs and rabbits. Fauci was impressed with the relative ease of splicing genes into this animal coronavirus, genes that could cause disease in humans.

Chapter 26

Gain of Function Research: Government Agencies Go Rogue

Let us look at the timeline of how the coronavirus was bioengineered into a major killer of humans:

1999, September 6th, Fauci began funding research at University of North Carolina, Chapel Hill to begin bioengineering the animal coronavirus.

2002, April 19th, Fauci designed a program in which Professor Ralph Baric PhD at the University of North Carolina Chapel Hill was instructed to commercially weaponize a naturally occurring spike protein toxin. This is the beginning of the criminal conspiracy and violates 18 USC § 175, 15 USC § 1-

3, and 15 USC § 8) Dr. Baric's expertise was discovering how to modify components of the coronavirus associated with human cardiomyopathy. NIAID Grants AI 23946 and GM63228 (leading to patent U.S. 7,279,327 "Methods for Producing Recombinant Coronavirus") was the NIH's first Gain-of-Function (GOF) project in which Dr. Baric created an "infectious, replication defective" clone of recombinant coronavirus. This work clearly defined a means of making a natural pathogen harmful to humans by manipulating the Spike Protein and other receptor targets. It was designed to specifically target human lung epithelium several months before the world's first outbreak in Asia. [36] [37] [38]

36

https://www.congress.gov/117/meeting/house/114270/documents/HHRG-117-GO24-20211201-SD004.pdf

[37]https://www.house.mi.gov/Document/?Path=2021_2022_session/committee/house/standing/workforce,_trades,_and_talent/meetings/2021-08-12-1/documents/testimony/Dr.%20Moehanid%20Talia.pdf
https://www.brown-watch.com/brownwatch-

2002-2004 Southeast Asian Respiratory Syndrome (SARS) began. The Chinese by then had been doing their own gain of function research with coronavirus and the cause of SARS therefore was either an accidental or a deliberate release of their bioengineered coronavirus. SARS had a minor effect in China; there were 8,469 cases and only 95 deaths. Fauci is in charge of all funding on research relating to the SARS virus in the United States.

2003, April 25th, The CDC filed patent 220,852 for the entire gene sequence of their bioengineered SARS coronavirus in violation of 35 USC 101 which prohibits the patenting of a naturally

---

news/2021/8/4/sdsds

[38] https://uploads-ssl.webflow.com/62f6c2ce87ee5b46474b4cf5/62f75221d95bf7724d4a6132_The-Criminal-Conspiracy-of-Coronavirus.pdf

occurring organism. The patent office found 99% of the CDC patent to be within the public domain, that is, what was believed by USPTO to be a natural coronavirus so the USPTO denied the patent. The CDC then bribed the USPTO by paying a filing fee and received the patent. The CDCs public relations department said they needed to create this patent so other virology labs could research what they knew to be their bioengineered virus. The CDC then paid another "special" fee to the USPTO to keep the patent private. If you want other labs to research a patented anything you do not pay a fee to keep the patent private.

2003, April 26th, The CDC applied for but did not receive two patents which covered what was actually a bioengineered SARS coronavirus patent 46,592,703p **and** a means of detecting the virus patent 776,521. If you own the patent of the gene and the PCR testing for that gene you have the ability to cause an infection and then the ability to identify it. This is a conflict of interest.

2003, April 28th, Sequoia Pharmaceuticals filed the patent 7,151,163 for a drug treatment for the SARS coronavirus, 3 days after the CDC patent was filed. How did Sequoia Pharmaceutical know about the CDC patent, it had not been granted yet and the CDC paid extra to have it be kept private, out of the public record! This is a violation of Ricoh laws, its racketeering, collusion and the definition of a criminal conspiracy. Later on Sequoia Pharmaceuticals was purchased by Pfizer Pharmaceuticals.

2005, July 5, DARPA, the defense advanced research program, expressed interest in SARS as a bioweapon. DARPA and MITRE (a private "national security" corporation), hosted a conference in which the intentions of the U.S. Department of Defense was explicit. In a presentation focused on "Synthetic Coronaviruses Biohacking: Biological Warfare Enabling Technologies", Dr. Baric presented the malleability of CoV(Coronavirus) as a biological warfare agent. Violating 18 USC § 175 and inducing the non-competitive market allocation (violating 15 USC § 8) for years to follow, Dr. Baric and The Department of Defense spent over $45 million in amplifying the toxicity of CoV and its chimeric (capable of changing form) derivatives. [39]

2008, July 15th, Ablynx Inc, now part of Sanofi Inc. filed a series of patents that targeted the polybasic cleavage site, the novel spike protein and the ACE2 receptor such as patent 9193780 that came into being after the gain of function moratorium, a violation of the law.

2008-2019, 73 patents by research facilities all over the world for SARS Cov2 bioengineered coronavirus were filed with USPTO.

---

[39] https://uploads-ssl.webflow.com/62f6c2ce87ee5b46474b4cf5/62f75221d95bf7724d4a6132_The-Criminal-Conspiracy-of-Coronavirus.p

2012, the Middle East Respiratory Syndrome began and showed up first in Saudi Arabia and later in 22 other countries. This second version of the bioengineered coronavirus was found in only 2,500 patients but the death rate went from 11% to 35%. The WHO estimated 554 deaths. During this coronavirus, epidemic ventilated patients died at a much higher rate than patients allowed to recover without this kind of medical intervention.

2015, the Congress passed a law that forbade scientific experimentation with "gain of function" research citing the dangers of these viruses getting loose in the public and causing pandemic proportion disease. This law, S.3012 — 117th Congress (2021-2022) was specifically aimed at preventing exactly what the Congress feared could happen if someone like Anthony Fauci continued this kind of work. Regardless of our Congressman trying to do the right thing, Fauci did something even more careless and foolish at this point and members of the Senate like Rand Paul M.D., and Roger

Marshall M.D. caught him doing it. He gave the virus to the Communist Chinese Party's Wuhan Virology Institute along with thousands and thousands of taxpayer dollars.

2016 Ralph S. Baric PhD, wrote a paper saying the you can make a lot of money with SARS Cov2.

2016, February 12th, Peter Daszak of the EcoHealth Alliance made the following statement which was recorded into the public record: "We need to increase public understanding of the need for clinical countermeasures, such as a pan corona vaccine, the key element is the media and the economics will follow the hype, we need to use that hype to our advantage, investors will respond if we see profit at the end of the process." [40]

Forum on Medical and Public Health Preparedness for Catastrophic Events; Forum on Drug Discovery, Development, and Translation; Forum on Microbial

---

[40] https://www.wnd.com/2021/06/fauci-funded-scientist-chinese-colleagues-created-killer-coronavirus/

Threats; Board on Health Sciences Policy; Board on Global Health; Institute of Medicine; National Academies of Sciences, Engineering, and Medicine. Rapid Medical Countermeasure Response to Infectious Diseases: Enabling Sustainable Capabilities through Ongoing Public- and Private-Sector Partnerships: Workshop Summary. Washington (DC): National Academies Press (US); 2016 Feb 12. 6, Developing MCMs for Coronaviruses. Available from: [41]

During this same year, Peter Dazak admitted that the NIH at Fauci's insistence, funded gain of function research at the Wuhan Virology Institute. He made the admission at a 2016 forum in a clip unearthed by the National Pulse.

In 2017, the gain of function ban was lifted but by this time the Wuhan Virology Institute in China already had the Fauci engineered bioweapon and continued their work to make it more virulent.

[41] https://www.ncbi.nlm.nih.gov/books/NBK349040/

In 2019, Fauci convinced NIH to give Wuhan Institute of Virology more money, $600,000 dollars over the next 6 years to continue the gain of function research on his coronavirus patents. [42]

2019, March, Moderna knew they would be first in line to produce a vaccine for the coronavirus so they applied for a patent for their vaccine claiming they needed to be ready for an accidental or deliberate release of SARS Cov2.

2019, November, In November 2019 – one month before the alleged "outbreak" in Wuhan, Moderna entered into a material transfer agreement – brokered by the Vaccine Research Center at NIAID to access Dr. Baric's Spike Protein data to commence vaccine development. In his own written

---

[42] https://www.factcheck.org/2021/05/the-wuhan-lab-and-the-gain-of-function-disagreement/
https://www.newsweek.com/dr-fauci-backed-controversial-wuhan-lab-millions-us-dollars-risky-coronavirus-research-1500741

statement obtained by the Financial Times, Dr. Barric refers to this agreement as being the foundation for the mRNA Moderna vaccine. [43] [44]

You can verify this information just like David Martin M.D. did by going to the United States Patent Office (USPTO) website. You will see 120 applications by Anthony Fauci for new patents on the bioengineered Coronavirus. Most of these patent requests were accepted, sometimes by USPTO agents under duress according to research uncovered by David Martin. [45]

---

[43] https://uploads-ssl.webflow.com/62f6c2ce87ee5b46474b4cf5/62f75221d95bf7724d4a6132_The-Criminal-Conspiracy-of-Coronavirus.pdf

[44] https://pubmed.ncbi.nlm.nih.gov/32756549/

[45] https://rumble.com/vk4znu-2021-jul-09-fauci-pharma-rico-usa-manufactured-illusion.-dr-david-martin-wi.html

2021 At a press conference, Fauci responded to a question that the gain of function research might have caused the pandemic that "the benefits outweigh the risks." [46] Please think about this for a minute. This statement made by the leader of the Coronavirus research effort in the United States claims that the resulting almost one million lives taken by his own bioengineered virus was a benefit that outweighed the risks of NOT doing the bioengineering research that he handed over to a regime in China that has a mission to overtake and absorb our very culture, country, assets and people! With a government official like Fauci in charge it's like giving the keys to the kingdom to a double agent from the Chinese Communist party. Did he Fauci ever show any remorse? No. As a matter of fact he has continuously hid behind his notoriety as being the head government Coronavirus expert to act as though he didn't care if people found out he

---

[46] https://www.nationalreview.com/news/fauci-argued-benefits-of-gain-of-function-research-outweighed-pandemic-risk-in-2012-paper/

was the puppet master behind the release of a bioweapon on his own people.

2021, October, U.S. Senator Roger Marshall, M.D. led a group of colleagues in introducing the *Viral Gain of Function Research Moratorium Act* to place a moratorium on all federal research grants to universities and other organizations conducting gain-of-function research and risky research on potential pandemic pathogens. This legislation is in response to the congressional inquiries and various media investigations revealing national security issues including federal agencies authorizing dangerous research with certain foreign entities that may have contributed to the COVID-19 pandemic. [47] [48]

---

[47] https://www.congress.gov/bill/117th-congress/senate-bill/3012/cosponsors?r=38&s=1
https://www.wsj.com/articles/covid-19-coronavirus-lab-leak-virology-origins-pandemic-11633462827

[48] https://www.marshall.senate.gov/wp-content/uploads/ROM21985.pdf

To share an insightful journalist's review of this issue, here is an excerpt from a recent Forbes magazine article by Steven Salzberg:

"After all the controversy over the past few years about gain-of-function research on viruses, especially the Covid-19 virus, I thought this kind of work was on hold, at least in the U.S. Indeed, the controversy grew so hot that NIH issued a statement in May of 2021 declaring that it would not support such work.

Nonetheless, some scientists continue to pursue gain-of-function work. In a new study, just released on the preprint server bioRxiv, a group of virologists at Boston University did the following. They took the Spike protein from the Omicron BA.1 strain of SARS-CoV-2 (that is the strain that spread throughout the world last winter, often slipping past the protection offered by vaccines) and combined it with an early 2020 strain of the Covid-19 virus.

This experiment gave them a brand-new, never-before-seen strain of Covid-19. Was it more deadly? You bet!

In their experiments, the BU scientists infected laboratory mice with the original Omicron virus, which caused "mild, non-fatal infection." Nevertheless, when they infected mice with their new, recombinant virus, which they called Omi-S, 80% of the mice died. To quote from their article:

"The Omicron S-carrying virus inflicts severe disease with a mortality rate of 80%."

Well, that is just great. Making matters worse, the researchers found that the new recombinant virus also replicated much faster in mice: "Omi-S-infected mice produced 30-fold more infectious virus particles compared with Omicron-infected mice." Yes, you read that right: Omi-S might grow

30 times faster than the garden-variety Omicron strain.

This, dear readers, is what we mean by "gain of function" research. The scientists took sequences from two different strains of the Covid-19 virus, one of which was relatively mild, and created a new strain that is far more infectious and far more deadly. As many scientists (and others) have pointed out, research like this carries great risks, foremost among them the chance that an accidental lab leak could create a new pandemic, killing millions of people." [49] [50]

---

[49] https://www.forbes.com/sites/stevensalzberg/2022/10/24/gain-of-function-experiments-at-boston-university-create-a-deadly-new-covid-19-virus-who-thought-this-was-a-good-idea/?sh=73195d6a5ca3

[50] https://childrenshealthdefense.org/defender/boston-university-scientists-engineering-viruses-labs-cola/

Fauci, Ralph Baric, Peter Daszak, and other CDC scientists over the last 20 years prepared the way for this pandemic and you and I paid for it with our tax dollars. I am sure you did not hear this on CNN or read about this in the New York Times or the Washington Post. The news media simply covered it up. Had reporters from any networks bothered to research the actions of these scientists, the causes of this pandemic would have been painfully obvious as early as January of 2020. Did you ever wonder why CNN, the New York Times, the Washington Post and other corporate media outlet reporters' rubber stamp whatever Fauci, the CDC and the WHO tell them? Could it be that the owners of most of these media outlets also own the large pharmaceutical companies like Pfizer, Moderna and Johnson & Johnson. Would that really surprise you?

OK diligent and courageous reader, now you understand how these scientists, led by Anthony Fauci, bioengineered the coronavirus along by inserting toxic genetic code sections over several years that led to the damages rendered to Covid-19 victims around the world. Your next question might be, "why would Fauci and scientists around the world do this". Again, to be very clear...they did it. There is no pretending they did not. The facts are there. They broke the laws of the United States of America.

You just saw them for yourself and there can be no question about their culpability because they left a trail for you to follow over a two-decade period. [51]

Well, you are not going to like the answer no matter how I present it so I'm going to just have to say it: Anthony Fauci and his colleagues are dangerous, blind sighted, arrogant, and careless scientists who have had no compunction endangering people around the world such that this bioweapon has culled millions of citizens from every country on earth.

[51] https://uploads-ssl.webflow.com/62f6c2ce87ee5b46474b4cf5/62f75221d95bf7724d4a6132_The-Criminal-Conspiracy-of-Coronavirus.pdf

Some people in both the scientific, medical and government communities believe Fauci is just dangerous and arrogant while others believe he has a depopulation agenda. Bill Gates clearly has a depopulation agenda. In December of 2021, he appeared in a TED talk where he said "the population of the world could be reduced by 20-15 percent by the use of vaccines." [52]

I am not a genius but when the fifth richest man in the world says directly on a forum of world intellectuals that vaccines can reduce our population, I have to take offense. He said it, they heard it, and now you just heard it. No beating around the bush. He had the chutzpah to say on camera vaccines are going to depopulate people into our future to reduce the human imprint and excessive consumption of resources. Wake up readers. Watch the video. Do not be afraid, it is not "misinformation". It is Bill Gates telling the world

[52] https://www.youtube.com/watch?v=CSRnPgncs3Q

he is coming for you with gene shots, the new jargon for what the so-called vaccine really is. Oh, you say, how could this be, Bill Gates is one of the good guys, right? [53]

Bill Gates' great grandfather is William H. Gates the first. He was a member of an organization called the American Eugenics Society. Their goal was to purify the genes of American citizens by forced sterilization of people deemed to be mentally handicapped, developmentally disabled, or injured in such a way that they were 'parasites on the taxpayer'. They also had a belief in controlling the population of the United States through sterilization of incarcerated Americans. Eventually members suggested the sterilization of Americans suffering from genetic diseases as well. [54] [55] The American

---

[53] https://www.youtube.com/watch?v=CSRnPgncs3Q

[54] https://heinonline.org/hol-cgi-bin/get_pdf.cgi?handle=hein.journals/iicl8&section=18

[55] https://heinonline.org/hol-cgi-

Eugenics Society was active from 1926 to 1972. Quietly sterilizations occurred right here in our own country! By the 1970s, the idea of forced sterilization was considered barbaric by many middle class Americans such that the society decided to reinvent their relationship with the public by renaming it. The membership simply began calling themselves "The Birth Control League" and later "Planned Parenthood". [56] I'm not making a political statement here about abortion, that's not the purpose of this book; I'm simply reporting factually about the new direction many eugenicists evolved in order to circumvent criticism by society and from the popular press. The American Eugenics Society had lost any moral high ground by 1972 and most states that had established policies

---

bin/get_pdf.cgi?handle=hein.journals/gwlr72&section=35

[56] https://heinonline.org/hol-cgi-bin/get_pdf.cgi?handle=hein.journals/uclawo19&section=10

for forced sterilization had stopped this decidedly unlawful and horrendous practice. [57] [58]

As much as you've been told the opposite by the corporate media, Anthony Fauci has NOT been a pillar of government professional conduct and a leader in the effort to stop the pandemic. Fauci has taken deplorable and dangerous risks over the last 20 years considering he was hired to protect the health of the American taxpayers who pay his salary. He has in truth, bioengineered the kind of virus Michael Crichton, Ian Fleming, Robin Cook and other apocalyptic fiction writers have written about. The difference is this man wants you to ignore the fact of his abuse of your trust, ignore his deliberate actions and believe he is a good guy

---

[57] https://www.thoughtco.com/forced-sterilization-in-united-states-721308#:~:text=1981,forced%20sterilization%20in%20U.S.%20history.

[58] https://www.newyorker.com/books/page-turner/the-forgotten-lessons-of-the-american-eugenics-movement

during this pandemic! The National Institute of Health spends thousands of your taxpayer dollars year after year on research. Who has been in charge during the last 38 years when it comes to viral infectious disease research? It is Fauci, acting as the director of the National Institute of Allergy and Infectious Disease, who has spent 50 billion dollars of taxpayer money on viral research, some of which went to fabricating this deadly virus. You might want to rethink your opinion of this fellow and his minions like Dr. Ralph Baric and other scientists at the NIH, the NIAID and the CDC. To check this out for yourself, simply contact the United States Patent Office. They recorded over 113 patents by Anthony Fauci M.D. on gain of function bioengineering of the natural Corona virus from 1998 to 2023. Better yet, watch the video of an interview of David Martin M.D. who owns the largest insurance company that underwrites science facilities that do research like Fauci was up to. During this interview David lays out the patents Fauci produced of his dangerous activities in the laboratories of Fort Dietrick, North Carolina. It becomes painfully clear after David's in-depth fact finding tour that Fauci is a self-absorbed criminal maniac who pushed his scientific staff to splice various genetic fragments such as the HIV genes and other toxic to humans over two decades. [59] From 2014-2017 Congress through the White House Office of Science Technology and the Department of Health and Human Resources forced a pause of gain of function research in the United States, this measure specifically directed at Fauci. [60] During these three years Fauci began his quest to give the research he had accumulated to date to the Chinese virology institute in Wuhan.

---

[59] : https://forbiddenknowledgetv.net/there-is-no-variant-not-novel-no-pandemic-dr-david-martin-with-reiner-fuellmich/

[60] https://en.wikipedia.org/wiki/Gain-of-function_research

Chapter 27

The Chinese Get Involved

Judy Mikovits has written some very powerful books on the way Gallo and Fauci have attempted to intimidate both Frank Ruscetti and her as he ran roughshod over these tireless honest, cautious virologists to reach his goals. This behavior led to Gallo's eventual theft of the credit for the discovery of the AIDs virus from Nobel Laureate Luc Montagnier. Judy wrote in the book "Ending Plague" that "Montagnier alleged the presence of elements of HIV, germ of malaria in the genome of coronavirus is "highly suspect", and it "could not have arisen naturally" The French researcher also alleged an "industrial accident" to have taken place in the Wuhan National Biosafety Lab. Is an accident the ONLY possibility for how the virus spread throughout China and the world? [61]

I ask you reader if you think the Chinese Communist Party considers depopulation as an ethical roadblock. Did you know that the population of China has been gradually shrinking over the last twenty years? The term one-child policy refers to a population planning initiative in China implemented between 1980 and 2015 to curb the country's population growth by restricting many families to a single child. That initiative was part of a much broader effort to control population growth that began in 1970 and ended in 2021, a half century program that included minimum ages at marriage and childbearing, minimum time intervals between births, heavy surveillance, and stiff fines

---

[61] Judy Mikovits et al, "End of Plague" (Children's Health Defense) page 256

for non-compliance. The program had wide-ranging social, cultural, economic, and demographic effects, although the contribution of one-child restrictions to the broader program has been the subject of controversy. **Harsh patriarchal attitudes** and a **cultural preference for sons** led to the abandonment of unwanted infant girls, some of whom **died** and others of whom were adopted abroad. Over time, this skewed the country's **sex ratio** toward men and created a **generation of "missing women"**. China currently has **37.17 million** more males than females. Consequently, one of the most lucrative and active retail businesses in Chinese major cities is the female sex doll store.

China's fertility rate has dropped over the years from the 2.1 birthrate required to replace the dying to only 1.15. China's population is projected to drop to 587 million in 2100. Is this an advantage to the Communist Party, the five unelected leaders who dictate the policies for its citizens? It definitely is! A smaller country is a much more "manageable" country, less protests of its policies, less money spent on domestic programs, more money to be spent on military and imperialist projects and the opulent lifestyles of the Communist Party members.

Whether the eventual release of the Fauci bio-engineered coronavirus in China in early 2020 was an accident or intentional, the result has been devastating. Currently the world has said goodbye to 6,630,000 souls dead from Covid-19. Maybe you want to reevaluate your opinion of Anthony Fauci and his 'team'.

Chapter 28

My Covid Look into the Future

I am a believer in scientists and physicians like myself who have come out in favor of the freedom for early treatment for Coronavirus infections and skepticism of the mRNA jab. In this chapter, I'm going to present current examples of people who have been active in reporting the effects of the Covid-19 vaccine. You are going to see examples of people in the medical field who over the last three years since the jab has been released, have changed their mind about the effectiveness and lack of safety of this vaccine and have come out of the closet to say so, some at the risk of their careers, jobs and incarceration.

By the way, I am not in favor of traditional influenza type vaccines. There have never been successful outcome studies for people who have chosen to receive vaccination over the last twenty years of the flu vaccines. Even worse, traditional flu vaccines are preserved with a mercury compound called thimerosal and even trace amounts of mercury go straight to the brain and increase the chances of Alzheimer's disease.

There is zero evidence for the effectiveness of Covid mRNA vaccines to date. Instead there is only evidence for the sudden death, heart damage, female system damage and others.

There are examples of:

- Increased fibrous clots in the blood of mRNA vaccinated corpses.
- Increased stillborn babies in mRNA vaccinated mothers.
- Increased deaths of mRNA vaccinated college and professional athletes.
- Increased deaths of mRNA vaccinated military soldiers.
- Increased deaths of mRNA vaccinated immune-comprised seniors.

Whistleblowers have been coming out of the woodwork to show the facts that are not being reported on the "Big Corporate News Outlets". Watch the film in the link below called "Died Suddenly". The evidence for the dangers of the vaccine is overwhelming. This film was written, directed, filmed and edited by Miller Skow and

Nicholas Stumphauser and produced by Stew Peters. [62]

This information is jaw dropping and well documented. I am going to present some major points to bring home the shared experience of these brave filmmakers, producers and whistleblowers.

The Embalmers:

Within 6 months from the January 2021, mass Covid-19 vaccination, embalmers from funeral homes all around the United States, Australia and Great Britain began to notice white fibrous clots or "structures" in the blood vessels of vaccinated people. Some of these clots were as long as three feet. The consensus is that these embalmers have not seen these clots prior to the mRNA vaccination. At a convention of embalmers in the United States over one hundred embalmers raised their hands

---

[62] https://screencast-o-matic.com/player/c3X0DKVU47u

when asked if they had seen these white fibrous clots in corpses vaccinated with mRNA.

When young athletes die suddenly, most of them will not be autopsied. The only evidence of the unnatural way in which they died will be observed by embalmers.

The Military Physicians

Lieutenant Colonel Teresa Long M.D. gave her testimony under the protection of Title 10 USC 1034, the whistleblower law, in September of 2022. She remarked on how insurance companies consider an increase of 10% of all-cause mortality in eighteen to sixty-four year olds to be a catastrophic event. One Indiana Life Insurance CEO was reported in "The Center Square" newspaper saying deaths are up 40% in eighteen to sixty-four year olds and he is just one insurance company in America but other companies are reporting similar statistics. Dr. Long testified, "I have never seen this litany of debilitating and potentially deadly medical conditions in soldiers. These conditions include strokes, transient ischemic attacks, pericarditis, myocarditis, erratic heartbeats, rapid onset progression of various cancers including testicular cancer, esophageal cancer, brain tumors, neuro-endocrine tumors, spinal tumors, thyroid dysfunction, multiple sclerosis, cognitive impairment, persistent severe insomnia, suppression of the immune system, unprovoked blood clots, avascular necrosis, liver dysfunction, menstrual irregularities and miscarriages."

It is therefore safe to estimate that this increase in deaths since the introduction of the vaccine is greater than the amount of deaths caused by Covid-19 in 2020. In other words, the vaccine is killing more people than the virus ever did.

Lieutenant Colonel Peter Chambers M.D., another military whistleblower, agrees with Dr. Long that the vaccine is killing our standing army. Dr. Long estimates that by 2027 "we will not have a viable military that can protect the United States."

At a hearing conducted by U.S. Senator Ron Johnson, attorney Tom Rems an attorney who represents medical members of the Department of Defense (DOD) gave testimony and presented declarations. These declarations exposed an increase of miscarriages by 300% over the 5-year average, an increase in cancer of 300% over the five-year average and increase in neurological conditions in pilots of 1000% since the beginning of the mRNA Covid 19 vaccinations began. This information was available on a DOD website called "DMED.gov and stands for "Defense Medical Epidemiological Database". Senator Johnson noticed the DOD and President Biden about these statistics demanding an investigation. Within 24 hours, the website was shut down until the "new and improved version" was put back online months later.

Dr. Ryan Cole

Dr. Ryan Cole M.D. a pathologist at his own private company in Idaho was one of the first physicians who saw an uptick in cancer following the mRNA vaccine. He spoke with various oncologist colleagues who all agreed this was occurring. He points out that the "Emergency use" granted pharmaceutical companies, allows them to put **anything** they want in these vials and the FDA isn't inspecting these facilities". Just recently, the Washington State Medical Board charged Dr. Cole with the following "Dr. Cole made numerous false and misleading statements related to COVID-19 and treated patients with COVID-19 or seeking to prevent getting COVID-19 in a manner that was beneath the standard of care". [63]

Of course, the standard of care established by the CDC and the FDA are the toxic drugs Remdesivir and the other two kidney toxic drugs Dexamethasone and Vancomycin. Oh and don't forget the useless ventilators. Dr. Cole resides in Idaho and his license has not been charged by the

---

[63] https://wmc.wa.gov/news/statement-charges-served-physician-license-ryan-cole

Idaho Board of Health. If they take his license away in Washington, it's hardly likely it will have a major impact on his ability to continue his work. Ryan Cole M.D. by the way completed a tour of the United State with Robert Malone M.D. to educate parents about the dangers of the Covid vaccine to their children. My wife and I were lucky enough to hear them in Gig Harbor Washington. These two tireless activists spoke on behalf of American children to bring clarity and truth to the evidence for the toxicity of this technology to standing room only crowd.

Normally when clinicians receive a typical childhood vaccine, the package insert unfolds into a very large document with detailed explanations of the product. When clinicians receive an mRNA vaccine, the package insert has nothing on it except: "intentionally left blank".

The Maternity Clinicians

Michelle Gibson R.N. is a nurse whistleblower from a major hospital in Fresno, California. She reports the following: "Before the vaccine there were one-two fetal demises (miscarriages, stillbirths, death after the 20th week of pregnancy) every two-three months. It was extremely rare. After the vaccine there were twenty-two fetal demises reported in one month and it was expected to increase each month".

James A.Thorp M.D. has been doing high risk obstetrics for years. "I see a vast number of patients a year. I don't know of any maternal fetal medical physician in this country that sees as many patients as I do by ultrasound. At one point I was on track to see 9,000 high risk O-B ultrasounds. I know what's going on and I've seen death and destruction like I've never seen before. Twelve hundred fold increases in menstrual abnormalities. When we get into pregnancies we see a substantial increase in miscarriages, birth defects, substantial risk of fetal cardiac arrhythmia, cardiac malformations, significant fetal growth slowing, significant reduction in amniotic fluid, fetal cardiac arrest (babies having heart attacks in the womb). The vaccine causes a significant inflammatory effect. Anything that causes inflammation in my field of expertise causes damage, injury, death and destruction in pregnancy. We've known that for half a century". [64]

On March 1st, 2021, the FDA released the first round of thousands of pages for review of Pfizer's Covid-19 vaccine. It was titled "5.3.6 Cumulative Analysis of Post Authorization Adverse Events". This document reported that 83% of pregnant women who got vaccinated wound up with a dead baby. In Hungary, the birth rate for 2022 fell by 20% exactly 9 months after the mass vaccination of the mRNA vaccine began. [65]

---

[64] https://worldcouncilforhealth.org/multimedia/adverse-events-pregnancy-fertility/

[65] https://phmpt.org/wp-content/uploads/2021/11/5.3.6-postmarketing-experience.pdf

Australia has seen a 70% decline in the birth rate, Taiwan 23% and the list goes on and on depending on the level of vaccination in that country.

None of the corporate think tanks are including the CDC evidence for the Covid-19 vaccination risk to pregnant women as a factor in the decline in fertility since the jab was released in 2021. Instead they dance around the elephant in the room by including other plausible reasons for the decline. Below is a summary of a paper presented by the PEW Charitable Trust on the subject:

- The pandemic economy has put off couples from having children
- Recent declines in immigration
- Recent declines in life expectancy
- The broader aging of the population [66]

[66] https://www.pewtrusts.org/en/research-and-analysis/issue-briefs/2022/12/the-long-term-decline-in-fertility-and-what-it-means-for-state-budgets

Sure, those reasons could be involved to a small extent but the point is to distract you from looking at the medical facts. The author is really saying, "Hey, the pandemic is the problem but not because it's **directly** affecting fertility, only because it's **indirectly** affecting fertility". Well, the CDC **is** saying the Covid-19 jab is **directly** affecting fertility but very few people are listening.

Angelia Desselle and many others have come forth with documented video of the seizure-like symptoms they experienced after taking the Covid-19 vaccine. Even Elon Musk has admitted on Twitter that he had neurological side-effects after getting a booster recently. Pfizer has doubled down to gaslight these victims of the jab by encouraging humorous fake seizure videos to mock these victims. Logically, there is no reason for a person previously trusting the protection offered by Pfizer to fake a seizure after administration of the jab. Angelia Desselle went on record as saying she was **not** anti-vaxxer prior to receiving the Covid jab. In fact, she presented proof that she had previously taken annual flu shots. [67]

Kirk Milhoan M.D. is a pediatric cardiologist from Maui, Hawaii. He was instrumental in encouraging early treatment with Ivermectin and Hydroxychloroquin in the summer of 2021. He was investigated by the Maui Board of Health but eventually absolved of any wrongdoing because from the beginning, he encouraged people to get vaccinated with the Covid jab. Just recently he appeared on a panel for Children's Health Defense TV with other anti-vaxers like Meryl Nass M.D. to expose the increase of myocarditis in young men given the vaccine. He shared how the CDC admitted that two hundred young males per millions of vaccinated suffered heart damage but these cases

[67] https://live.childrenshealthdefense.org/chd-tv/shows/good-morning-chd/thankspfizer-the-mass-gaslighting-of-angelia-desselle/?utm_source=email&utm_medium=salsa&utm_campaign=CHD+TV&utm_term=chdtv&eType=EmailBlastContent&eId=5938c0e8-456c-4399-ae86-08b0a6f43f47

were only those that went to the hospital. He reported another myocarditis study from Thailand where the researchers showed 20,000 per million young men showed heart damage. Quite the disparity wouldn't you say? It's always nice to see a physician like Dr. Milhoan who went along originally with the Big Pharma Covid-19 vaccine party line, gradually reevaluate his position on mRNA safety. [68]

Chapter 29

The Good News

[68] https://www.google.com/search?q=kirk+milhoan+md+covid&newwindow=1&rlz=1C1GCEA_enUS1043&sxsrf=AJOqIzXtUfPeAjrxXy3-6H_oibu6GIp-gA%3A1675202308574&ei=BI_ZY9HSlv2H0PEP2OCDqAc&ved=0ahUKEwjR5J305vL8AhX9AzQIHVjwAHUQ4dUDCBA&uact=5&oq=kirk+milhoan+md+covid&gs_lcp=Cgxnd3Mtd2l6LXNlcnAQAzIFCCEQoAEyBQghEKABOgUIABCABDoGCAAQFhAeOgUIIRCrAjoICCEQFhAeEB1KBAhBGAFKBAhGGABQ6AJY5Q1glhFoAXAAeACAAV-lAawDkgEBNpgBAKABAcABAQ&sclient=gws-wiz-serp#ip=1

As of January 2023, 71.8% of the world's population has been Covid-19 vaccinated but the numbers are dropping. As of December 14th 2022 85% of Americans have had at least one Covid-19 jab but more and more are declining further injections. Many Americans who took the jab in 2021 did so to keep their jobs or travel but now in early 2023 they are rethinking continuing with the CDC's suggested program of boosters as more and more evidence surfaces of the dangers. Parents are rethinking allowing their children to get the jab. Adults are discouraging their family and friends to get the jab and the word is spreading. The CDC's own website reports that fourteen percent of Americans today do not trust the Covid-19 vaccine. Let that sink in. In January of 2021 people were lining up all over America and couldn't wait to get stuck with at least eighty-five percent getting one Covid-19 shot. Three years later fourteen percent do not trust the vaccine. Nowadays, the CDC is one unhappy government agency. I call that progress: [69]

The confidence level varies by state. Many of the red states show less enthusiasm for the Covid-19 jab than the blue states. One such state is Florida whose governor has by far spearheaded the opposition to mandatory vaccination all along. Just recently CNN reported the following: "Amid rising Covid-19 cases across the US, Florida Republican Governor Ron DeSantis is pushing to permanently ban coronavirus vaccine and face mask mandates in his state. Governor DeSantis, a vocal Covid-19 skeptic, signed measures in 2021 that made Florida the first state in the country to threaten businesses with fines if they required workers to get a Covid-19 vaccine. In addition to proposing permanent bans on mask and vaccine mandates, DeSantis also wants to prevent doctors from losing their medical licenses if they stake out positions that contradict

---

[69] https://www.ncbi.nlm.nih.gov/pmc/articles/PMC8202656/

medical consensus. This comes as medical experts have noted a national decline in childhood vaccination numbers. Among several reasons, experts say misinformation and disinformation around Covid-19 vaccines may have seeded doubt in other vaccines". Thanks, CNN, we know how to translate the word "disinformation", when you and the press sycophants use it, it means "truth-sayers". [70] I was sorry to hear the Governor DeSantis dropped out of the race for the presidency. DeSantis and RFK Jr. are now the only presidential candidates that NEVER trusted Fauci, the CDC and Biden to do the right thing when the Covid virus showed up in our fair country. Former president Trump stood by Fauci and the vaccine from the beginning.

Other state governors are following suit with DeSantis. One such man is Governor Greg Abbott of Texas. This Covid-19 policy statement comes

---

[70] https://mail.google.com/mail/u/0/#inbox/FMfcgzGrcFhRtQclLwbWRrQmDGcCbGCL

directly from the governor's website: "While the CDC's Advisory Committee on Immunization Practices has recommended adding routine COVID-19 immunization to the 2023 immunization schedules for adults and children, that recommendation does not create any federal vaccination mandate. Texas has no state or local COVID-19 immunization requirements. Pursuant to Governor Abbott's Executive Order GA-39, which has been in effect since August 25, 2021, no government entity in Texas can mandate the COVID-19 vaccine". [71]

Those of you who have shown the courage to read this book to this point can take action. Whether you have been vaccinated or not, reduce the level of inflammation in your body by reducing your exposure to carcinogens. All animal food is either a Group 1 or Group 2 carcinogen. Bacon, hot dogs, sausage, lunch meats are Group 1 carcinogens.

---

[71] https://www.dshs.texas.gov/covid-19-coronavirus-disease-2019/covid-19-vaccine-information

Don't take my word for it, the U.S. Department. Agriculture reported this finding several years ago. This means that **all** foods listed in Group 1 **definitely** cause cancer, there is no question. All other animal foods such as beef, pork, chicken, turkey, fish, seafood, eggs and dairy products are Group 2 carcinogens, that is, they **probably** cause cancer.

Cancer is the final insult to the body caused by long term inflammation. You wouldn't drink toxic chemicals or eat toxic mushrooms so at least reduce if not eliminate toxic food. Doing this will give your detoxification organs a huge benefit by increasing their ability to protect all your organs and tissues from inflammation.

Most Americans have been eating beef, pork, lamb, poultry, fish, cheese, cottage cheese, yogurt and eggs several times a day for the last about 150 years since the industrial revolution invented mass production of animal food. The typical **pre-industrial** revolution Western diet was based on grains, legumes, vegetables, fruits, nuts, and seeds with only occasional animal food meals as a treat.

Back then only the very rich could afford daily animal food products. A study of the fossilized remains of the Pharaohs all the way to studies of modern omnivores reveals the truth that degenerative diseases are caused by excess animal food. We live longer due to easier access to clean water, sanitation, safer childbirth and emergency rooms but unless we die quicker we spend our senior years suffering from inflammation. People need to get back to their original diet.

This program brings you into a transformative lifestyle that acts as therapy reinventing your eating habits not only to help reverse your conditions but to give you more energy to exercise and less physiologic stress to enhance your sleep. It has been used successfully to treat most chronic, degenerative conditions from cardiovascular disease and cancer to arthritis, fibromyalgia, multiple sclerosis and others.

Our original diet of breast milk or formula released 85% of its calories from carbohydrate, only 5% from protein and 10% from fat. These low-protein first foods will double the size of a newborn in only six months! Newborns are on a low protein, low fat diet and yet they build muscle and bone easily. Research on plant based diet-mothers has demonstrated that after weaning, when the infant is put on a diet similar to breast milk it will thrive greater than all infants on animal food-based diets. By the time an infant reaches about twenty-five years of age, the body begins the slow path to transition (death). Once the child is a young adult if they avoid excess protein and fat they will live physically healthier and longer.

Because food isn't as easy to digest as breast milk, this diet is designed to have twice as much protein as the infant gets, 10% of its calories from protein not 5%, 10% from fat and 80% from carbohydrates. Of the carbohydrates, most of the calories come from starch. Starch releases sugar slowly into the blood at only one calorie per gram, even for people challenged with diabetes and hypoglycemia. The Standard American Diet (S.A.D) of 2 servings of animal protein a day provides 30% from protein and 30% from fat but only 40% of its calories from carbohydrates. An 80-10-10 carb, protein, fat diet gives the body the best chance to stay optimally healthy or restore health.

Fat contains nine calories per gram and any extra fat above the 10% you would eat on an 80-10-10 diet ends up increasing fat in the body. ALL oils and butter are refined foods and add additional calories and acidity. Excess fat breaks down into fatty acids. Excess protein breaks down into excess amino acids. All this excess acidity creates inflammation in the cells of the liver, kidneys, heart, blood vessels, muscles, joints, nervous system, and brain.

Refined sugar contains four calories per gram while fruit releases only two calories per gram due to the water, fiber, enzymes, and phytochemicals present in these antioxidant and anti-inflammatory rich treats. Potatoes, brown rice, quinoa, lentils and other starches release only one calorie per gram.

Autopsy studies on typical young Americans by age twenty-five show 50% fat (including cholesterol) blocking their arteries because **excess** fat leads to gradual deposits of plaque which leads to clotting events to the heart and brain as the person ages. Clogging of arteries is usually systemic and leads not just to heart attacks and strokes but back pain, shoulder pain, dementia, erectile dysfunction and other disorders due to decreased blood flow. As excess fat coats muscle cells, insulin receptors are blocked and diabetes begins. Excess sugar doesn't lead to diabetes; it feeds yeast, bacteria, fungus, parasites, worms and other bugs which accelerate diabetes and all other degenerative diseases.

An important part of this program is to reduce as close to zero as possible added salt, oil and sugar (S.O.S.). Eating more than the adequate salt, available in the Whole Food, Plant Based, Starch Based, 80-10-10 diet unnecessarily stimulates appetite. Then, adding refined oil and sugar as mentioned are toxic and lead to degenerative disease and suffering.

This lifestyle is NOT a vegan diet because you are allowed to eat animal protein on special occasions, limiting yourself to twice a month which your body can recover from. It's best to begin "cheating" after you have healed yourself from your big challenges, the silent killers, heart disease, strokes, cancer, osteoporosis, and auto-immune conditions.

The Whole Food, Plant Based, 80-10-10 lifestyle will provide you with a lifetime free from degenerative disease. Are you committed to spending the last twenty years of your life juggling medical doctor and alternative doctor appointments from self-induced suffering? Instead of eventually having to swallow piles of pharmaceuticals or nutriceuticals to juggle the effects of your various symptoms you will be able to spend **quality** time with hobbies, projects and the people you love.

To further your education, please click on links to these other physicians and experts who are trim, healthy and strong and have been curing illness for decades with lifestyle changes alone:

Mic. the Vegan humorous weekly short science based videos available on YouTube.com

John McDougall MD   www.drmcdougall.com
Alan Goldhamer DC www.healthpromoting.com
Michael Klaper MD   www.doctorklaper.com

Dean Ornish MD   www.deanornish.com

Caldwell Esselstyn MD   www.dresselstyn.com

T. Colin Campbell PhD www.nutritionstudies.com

Joel Fuhrman M.D. www.drfuhrman.com

Garth Davis M.D. www.proteinaholic.com
Neil Barnard M.D. www.nutritionMD.org
Michael Greger M.D. http://drgreger.org

VIDEOGRAPHY Streamable on NetFlix or Amazon Prime

Forks over Knives, What the Health, Cowspiracy, Mad Cowboy

The best way to give this lifestyle a reasonable try is to work with a plant-based physician who can coach you on the proper way to give this lifestyle the two weeks therapeutic trial it deserves while custom tailoring it to your specific condition issues.

Whole Food, Plant Based Meals:

These meals are designed for people on the go; they take five-ten minutes to prepare.

Eat the vegetables, then the starch and end with fruit.

Eat until you are full with only sips of water; add no salt, oil or sugar (SOS).

All meals are made from whole foods, are plant based, the calories come predominantly from starch, comply with the 80-10-10 system, and contain only the salt, oil and sugar that occur naturally in foods. The great taste comes from recipes and the spices.

Day 1

BREAKFAST: Oatmeal with Almond slices, Blueberries

1 cup of water
1 cup of quick organic steel cut oats
bring water to a boil
add in oats
let boil at a rapid rate till gruel consistency
pour into large bowl add **1 tbsp. almond slices,**

½ cup blueberries and 1 tsp cinnamon
add 1/4 cup almond, rice or soy milk and mix

LUNCH: Baked Potatoes, Spring Greens spiced with Arugula

After Breakfast, place 2 medium red, or 2 white or 1 large Russet potato in the oven for 65 minutes. Use an oven with a timer that shuts off when it's done.
When it's time for lunch the potato will be cooled down ready to eat.
In a large bowl place a good portion of Spring Greens and Arugula.
Add enough water to cover and let it soak in for one minute. Decant the water.
Eat FIRST before the potato…can be eaten plain or mixed or dipped in any plain or fruit flavored white or dark balsamic vinegar or vinegar of your choice.
Cut potatoes into wedges and dip in hummus. Buy a hummus with 3.5 or less grams of fat per serving

and as little salt as possible or make it from my recipe.

DINNER: Brown rice and Salad

Make a Salad with your favorite vegetables using only vinegars of your choice and eat first. Then open a pre-cooked brown rice packet and place contents in a medium skillet with 2 tbsp. water and heat until warmed to your desire. You can mix in hummus, nut butter, any unsweetened mustard, hot sauce…just don't do them all together please. Most packets contain about 450-500 calories which is perfect for most middle-aged and senior adults. Eat more or less as needed.

DAY 2

BREAKFAST: Oatmeal with Almond slices, Raspberries

1 cup of water
1 cup of quick organic steel cut oats
bring water to a boil
add in oats
let boil at a rapid rate till gruel consistency
pour into large bowl add **1 tbsp. almond slices, ½ cup raspberries** and 1 tsp cinnamon
add 1/4 cup almond, rice or soy milk and mix

LUNCH: Amy's Soup, Toast and Fruit
1 can Amy's low salt lentil, split pea, black bean or minestrone, plain or warmed
grain bread you tolerate toasted or not with/without cashew-soft butter
fruit of your choice

DINNER: Organic Vegan Burger

Organic soy protein free vegan burger (made without dairy or eggs)

Whole grain bun or sliced bread, tomato, pickles, lettuce
Hummus and/or soft cashew butter, mustard, unsweetened, unsalted ketchup
Fruit of your choice

DAY 3

BREAKFAST: Oatmeal, Pumpkin Seeds and Blueberries

1 cup of water
1 cup of quick organic steel cut oats
bring water to a boil
add in oats
let boil at a rapid rate till gruel consistency
pour into large bowl add **1 tbsp. pumpkin seeds, ½ cup blueberries** and 1 tsp cinnamon
add 1/4 cup almond, rice or soy milk and mix

LUNCH: Curry Almond, Rice, Quinoa

½ pre-cooked rice or rice and quinoa packet (warms up in 1 minute)
1 tbsp. almond slices, 1 tsp raisins, 1 tsp curry powder
2 celery stalks, 1 carrot, 1/3 cucumber, sliced
Hummus-oil free (see recipe)
fruit of your choice

dip veggies in hummus and eat first filling the stomach 1/3 full
warm up the grain in a tbsp. of water for 2 minutes adding almonds, raisins, curry

DINNER: Garlic Mashed Potatoes and Salad

Salad with tomato, cucumber, lettuce
Thinned hummus or cashew soft butter or both or Bragg's Braggberry salad dressing
Boiled of baked potatoes, mashed
Raw or granulated garlic and onion cooked into the potatoes
Fruit of your choice

DAY 4

BREAKFAST: Oatmeal with walnuts, raspberries and cinnamon

1 cup of water
1 cup of quick organic steel cut oats
bring water to a boil
add in oats
let boil at a rapid rate till gruel consistency
pour into large bowl add **1 tbsp. walnuts,
½ cup raspberries** and 1 tsp cinnamon
add 1/4 cup almond, rice or soy milk and mix

LUNCH: Burrito with rice and vegetables

Whole grain tortilla that you tolerate
½ cup brown rice
Cilantro, tomato, lettuce, olives, avocado as desired
Fresh salsa or bottled hot sauce

warm up the tortilla on a dry frying pan, both sides and warm the rice
add all ingredients into tortilla and fold
Fruit of your choice
DINNER: Steamed vegetables and black beans

Steam fresh broccoli, chopped onion, red bell pepper, mushrooms
Mix in 1 tbsp cashew butter and 1 tbsp hummus
½ can black beans and ½ can corn with bread or crackers you tolerate
Fruit of your choice

DAY 5

BREAKFAST: Hash browns

1 ½ cups of shredded potato from scratch or rehydrated
One spray of oil
Banana

Spray large skillet with Pam or other spray oil (no calories)
Fry potatoes until golden on each side
Fruit of your choice

LUNCH: Black bean tacos

Soft Corn Tortillas
Cooked Black beans, mashed
Cashew Soft butter
Lettuce, tomato, olives

Warm up the tortilla on a dry frying pan, spread on the cashew butter and layer with beans, lettuce, olives and tomato

Fruit of your choice

DINNER: Dr. Rick's Famous Fresh Salsa Meal

6 medium or 4 large tomatoes chopped small, ½ green bell pepper chopped small
1 entire bunch of cilantro chopped fine, ½ medium onion chopped small
6 limes, juiced, 1 can low salt black beans (less than 100mg)
1 can low salt cut corn or 1 large corn on the cob cut, 1 tsp cumin, ½ tsp black pepper

Mix all ingredients and Eat with low salt blue or yellow baked tortilla chips till full
Fruit of your choice

DAY 6

BREAKFAST: Oatmeal with Almond slices, Blueberries

1 cup of water
1 cup of quick organic steel cut oats

bring water to a boil
add in oats
let boil at a rapid rate till gruel consistency
pour into large bowl add **1 tbsp almond slices, ½ cup blueberries** and 1 tsp cinnamon
add 1/4 cup almond, rice or soy milk and mix

LUNCH: Jack Fruit Reuben Sandwich

2 slices of whole grain bread
1 tbsp of vegan thousand island dressing
1 cup of jack fruit
½ cup sauerkraut
Spread thousand island on the bread, sauerkraut on one side, jack fruit on other
Combine both sides and place on oil sprayed skillet, brown and serve with fruit

DINNER: Dr. Rick's famous Pasta Salad

Farfalle (bowtie) pasta (regular) 2 cups, cooks in 11 minutes
Tomatoes, chopped fine, 2 cups
Cucumber, chopped fine, 1 cup
Bell pepper, any color, chopped fine, 1 cup
Cilantro, chopped, ½ bundle
Olives, Kalamata, chopped, ½ cup
Vinegar
Mix ingredients together in a large bowl and serve
Fruit of your choice

Day 7

BREAKFAST: Whole Grain Pancakes

1.5 cups whole grain flour of your choice
2 tsp aluminum free baking powder
1 cup (2.5 medium) mashed bananas
¼ egg replacer mixed with ¼ cup water until frothy
1 cup nondairy milk
1 tablespoon prune puree or applesauce

Mix flour and baking powder in a bowl and set aside

Mix the rest of the ingredients, add the dry ingredients and mix well

Place ¼ cup of batter on medium high skillet; use one spray of oil if necessary

Top with applesauce or bit of maple syrup

LUNCH: Mango Relish Rice

½ pre-cooked brown rice/quinoa packet
1 tsp Patak's mango relish (mild/medium or hot)
½ cup zucchini, ¼ cup bell pepper, ½ broccoli heads

Steam veggies 6 minutes, warm rice with 1 tbsp water, combine with relish

Fruit of your choice

DINNER: Pizza!!!

Whole Grain no oil Crust see YouTube.com [72]
or Cauliflower no oil Crust see YouTube.com [73]

[72] (https://youtu.be/v3cZ5wJ8Y9Q)

Low salt, no oil pasta sauce
1 cup cashews
½ cup chopped yellow bell pepper
½ - ¾ cup water
Toppings of your choice, spread pasta sauce on the crust
Blend cashews, yellow bell, and water to make a thick spread
Place toppings on top and bake for 15-20 minutes

Notes:

- Eating until you are full activates stretch receptors to signal the brain to reduce your appetite so you won't snack in between meals; if you forget to eat enough it's ok to have a bit more food midmorning or mid-afternoon but not before bed
- This is a no S.O.S program…no added salt, oil or sugar, just what comes in food.

---

[73] https://www.youtube.com/watch?v=yVZ7hXt3Ya8

- No added oil or fat of any kind. THE FAT YOU EAT IS THE FAT YOU WEAR.
- No added salt as just ¼ tsp salt contains 581 mg of sodium. Sodium is an appetite stimulant and raises blood pressure.
- No added sugar…refined sugar, as opposed to whole food sugar as in fruit, is an appetite stimulant by feeding intestinal bugs that stimulate appetite for sweets.
- Use spices of your choice to make food taste better they have zero calories.
- If you have to decide between non-organic plant food and organic animal food, always go with commercially grown plant food as even grass fed, free range animal food is more toxic to the digestive tract, liver, kidneys, immune system, brain, and energy. The exception is wheat containing products which MUST be eaten organic due to the

high levels of toxic herbicides like Round-Up.
- Costco and Sam's club have bulk steel cut oats in a five lb bags
- Costco and Sam's club have bulk organic soups and pre-cooked brown rice packets. They often come with other grains like quinoa which adds more flavor.
- Costco and Sam's club have bulk organic almond milk, rice and soy milk.
- Bragg's Braggberry and Tropical salad dressings have a mild sweet whole fruity flavor for a low salt and oil free salad dressing.
- Cholula and Syracha are my favorite hot sauces for when I don't have fresh salsa.
- Avoid processed soy protein, AKA isolated soy protein, soy protein, soy powder, and TVP as they triple the IGF-1 which leads to cancer. Soy milk, tempeh and tofu products not only don't increase IGF-1 but help with hormone balance to both sexes.

- You can have ½ tsp of ANY sweetener twice a day in tea or coffee and have 2 squares of dark chocolate per day if you can do that without binging, but if you're like many and you cannot, just let it go while you concentrate on eating lots of tasty, starchy foods you've denied yourself for so long...spiced up as you like!
- If you must eat at a restaurant because you're out of town or it's a special occasion see the youtube.com video below for ideas on what to order: "Dr. **McDougall eating out**": [74]
- If you are invited to a restaurant, eat a good meal before you go and have tea, decaf, salad with vinegar or cooked veggies while there; don't let others pressure you into getting as overweight or chronically dysfunctional as they are.

---

[74] https://www.youtube.com/watch?v=1bfloOiSrSQ

Cashew Nut Butter

1 cup raw cashew pieces
½ cup water

Blend
Pour into container with lid and refrigerate
Shelf life is two weeks

Best to use at least a Ninja blender at ~$80 or Vitamix or Blendtec ~$300-400.
This is a very sweet butter.
You may want to cut it with almonds or use them alone.
You can add ⅓ cup of some veggies but this cuts the shelf life down to 5-7 days.
It thickens a bit in the fridge.

Thinning it with water makes a nice salad dressing. It adds a lot to steamed vegetables

Green Drink Recipe (120 calories)

Water 4 oz
Blueberries ½ cup
Banana ½
Apple ½
Organic vanilla protein powder 1 tablespoon or half scoop
Greens (kale, spinach, chard) 2 cups or large Blend till smooth, tastes mildly sweet
You can swap or mix artichoke spears, celery, and lettuce for Greens

All these items can be purchased organically at Costco.
The Brand name at Costco is ORGAIN organic VANILLA protein powder
Please go out of your way to buy organic if you can, you don't want to drink a health smoothie

containing Roundup (glyphosate) and other chemicals.

Hummus Oil Free

This easy delicious hummus starter can be varied using different spices and vegetables.

1 can low salt garbanzo beans AKA chickpeas
2 heaping Tbsp sesame butter
2 Tbsp fresh or frozen (not chemically stabilized=quite toxic) lemon juice
2 cloves fresh garlic

Blend, pour into container with lid and keep refrigerated
Shelf life on week
Excellent by itself
Wal-Mart and Costco sells organic low salt, less than 200 mg beans

Corn Grits Recipe

½ cup Bob's **Organic** Corn Grits/Polenta
1 ½ cup water
Healthy margarine of your choice 1 tsp
Salt, a few shakes
Season with anything you like

Boil the water.
Stir in the grits slowly and turn the heat down by 1/3
Stir occasionally for 3-4 minutes
Add the salt, margarine and seasoning

This cooked breakfast grain makes a nice alternative to oatmeal
I eat it once or twice a week instead of oatmeal

You can learn more about how to eat a healthier diet and physiologically why our bodies are not made to eat meat by getting my book: "First Do No Harm", a practical guide to plant based diet and medicine available from Amazon.com.

Chapter 30

The Good News: Supplements I Recommend for both Unvaccinated and Vaccinated

People who are Covid Unvaccinated: Take a few simple supplements not available easily in the diet once in the morning:

1. Vitamin B12 as methylcobalamin 1,000 mcg taken once daily. It is not easy to get 1,000 mcg in many diets and important for energy systems in the body.
2. Boron 3 mg taken once daily is a mineral deficient in almost all U.S. soils. It's

necessary for bone density through proper calcium maintenance.

3. Copper 2 mg, taken once daily is a mineral deficient in almost all U.S. soils. It's very important for immune function, joint repair and cardiovascular health.

4. MSM 1,000 mg taken once daily is a mineral deficient in all U.S. soils. It's a sulfur mineral donor that is effective if made by the special process developed by the discoverer Stanley Jacobs MD. It helps the body produce glutathione, the body's most powerful and abundant antioxidant. It's also a prerequisite for glucosamine sulfate and chondroitin sulfate the constituents of joint cartilage.

5. Vitamin D3 10,000 units taken once daily if you live in Northern states or don't get enough sun in southern states. It is an important immune system and bone building nutrient.

6. Liposomal Vitamin C, 1000 mg once daily provides extra antioxidant protection from environmental, food, water and geo-engineering contamination.

Remember to take all supplements with some food if you believe you might react to these concentrated nutrients.

People who are Covid-19 vaccinated or concerned about shedding:

Covid-19 Vaccinated people should take the supplements recommended in the list above and an extra one listed below to protect them from the short and long term effects of receiving a piece of mRNA genetic code they have no way of knowing when and if it will ever leave their system. People concerned about receiving the spike protein exhaled by vaccinated people (shedding) should take it as well:

Nattokinase 100 mg, 2,000 FU, which digests spike proteins and blood clots. This supplement is actually an enzyme, a very large molecule that digests spike proteins and clots that form from high blood pressure acting on cholesterol-fatty-calcium plaques that the line the arteries of the average American.

Supplement plan for Covid-19 vaccinated people:

1. Vitamin D-10,000 units 1 cap in the morning
2. Vitamin B12 (methylcobalamin) 1,000 mcg 1 cap in the morning
3. Boron 3mg 1 cap in the morning
4. Copper 2 mg 1 cap in the morning
5. MSM 1,000 mg, 3 caps morning and evening
6. Liposomal vitamin C 1,000 mg 1 cap in the morning
7. Nattokinase 100 mg, 2,000 FU 1 cap morning and evening

The cost of this program varies by source but I've been able to get them for less than $65 per month. Do you have to take the first four suggested for unvaccinated people? Yes because they allow the body to work properly in the first place. Do you have to take the Nattokinase recommended for vaccinated people? Who can say? There are very few controlled studies with these products for the Covid-19 vaccinated population as it has come along so fast. This protection is just as experimental so there is no good answer to that question. If you can afford it you should take all of them because your life is valuable to you is it not? You can't function well when you're sick with Covid symptoms and you certainly can't help your loved ones if you can't function well.

Some of them are not easy to obtain at a reasonable price and some aren't manufactured by well sourced companies. If you have any problem obtaining them, email me at nhcdirector@gmail.com

Chapter 31

The Future of the New mRNA Vaccine Technology

Modern medicine that began in the early 1900s has been promoted by Big Government. As it grew, modern medicine turned into Big Pharma and has brought the world many important benefits to **saving** lives in the emergency room and the surgical suite from life threatening infections to accidents and injuries.

Now it seems as if just recently, Big Pharma and Big Government are more interested in **taking** lives for some reason. We have just observed our own government sanction its head infectious disease scientist to release a new disease and then watched the same government give the nod to Big Pharma. Many Americans believe that Big Pharma has become a pharmaceutical cartel. Now this cartel seems to have conspired to create a scary new vaccine that injures and kills people who take it.

What about the people that survived the vaccine? There is evidence that Big Pharma released this harmful vaccine alongside placebo saline doses. This might have been done to confuse the population into continuing to accept the vaccine because if EVERYONE who took the vaccine suffered injury or death, no one would ever take it.

Chapter 32

What you can do about all this

Maybe it's time to take real Congressional action to curb both the purveyors of new unusual diseases and the genetic time bombs they use to "treat" them with.

You can encourage your family and friends to share the names of the U.S. Senators and Congressional Representatives listed in this book that are investigating Fauci et.al and Big Pharma for their criminal activities. You can donate to their campaign funds. You can write your Senators and Congressmen asking them to pay attention to the evidence for the corruption of the CDC and the NIH regarding both the Covid-19 virus origin and the rushed development of the vaccine.

Don't be a victim. Spread the word.

Epilog

Both of my attorneys told me they have never heard of a case like this before ever going to trial. They were surprised that I wasn't given a warning by the FDA or the FTC first which is the usual protocol in their experience. They were shocked at the apparent collusion between the judges and the prosecutors to secure a conviction. Over 2 million taxpayer dollars has been spent on my case so far.

On October 8th, 2022, just a week after I was released from the Federal Prison Camp at Sheridan and sent to the half-way house, the 9th Circuit Court of Appeals "fast tracked" the hearing of my case. My wife Rose was able to stream the hearing from a computer. I was just walking through the door of the half-way house and had no access to a computer yet.

During the hearing my wife explained to me when I got home later for a 48 hour pass that one of the 3 judges asked the prosecutor if she shipped oatmeal to a friend across state lines and said it could help with cholesterol in a note in the package, could she be prosecuted by the 21 USC 331 statute? The prosecutor responded yes. This observation by my attorneys seemed promising to our case and both my wife and I were a bit encouraged, just not for the long wait that ensued.

It took an entire year of this "fast tracked" Court of Appeals hearing for the three judges to return a "conviction as stands" reply which meant my conviction would not be overturned. Undeterred, my attorneys contacted me on October 17th, 2023 about our next step. They sent the request for a review of the case to the rest of the 9th Circuit Appeals Court judges. By this time, my lead attorney had quit the Federal Public Defenders office and gone into private defense practice. On February 22, 2024 I was called by my remaining attorney who informed me that the other 9th Circuit federal appellate judges had stood with the original three who had upheld the conviction.

At this point there was only one last step: submission of this case to the Supreme Court of the United States (SCOTUS). While any federal conviction must be heard by a Federal Appeals Court, over one thousand cases are submitted every year to the Supreme Court but only about one hundred or so are ever considered by this lofty judicial body.

I got a call from my attorney in May who informed me that the Supreme Court had decided not to review my case. The Supreme Court in my opinion couldn't risk taking my case. Think of the blowback on the FDA and Big Pharma.

I've decided to publish this book now that all the conventional legal doors have closed to me. But just to keep my cheerfulness a bit better, there is one last Hail Mary Pass possibility. A few weeks ago in early July the Supremes released a decision to overturn a 1980s decision call Chevron Deference. At that time, SCOTUS passed a decision in favor of an environmental group NRDC (National Resource Defense Council) verses Chevron Oil. Regardless of how you feel about the environment, in this decision, the ability of the courts to determine how congressional laws are interpreted was given to agencies like EPA, FDA, FBI and others and taken away from the courts. With this Chevron Deference decision, SCOTUS has decided that the courts should determine how to interpret Congressional laws. The idea here is that many agencies have been running amok, writing their statutes like 22USC331 which convicted me of an action that was not only harmless but lead to protecting the health and lives of Americans.

I now have a paralegal friend. I really like this guy and he's very smart. He has offered to take action on my case with this potentially new SCOTUS decision in hand. He has advised me that it's quite the long shot so all we can do is hope.

In this world there are people who wake up every day, go to work, come home to dinner, a beer or glass of wine and the TV news, take their annual vacation and see a movie once a month. Only half of these adults vote in federal and state elections. When Covid-19 came along sixty-five percent opened their arms and accepted this briefly tested "vaccination" with trepidation and hope in their hearts and minds.

After three years of post vaccination history, these same people are waking up to the evidence for the possibility that the crime reported in this took place. That is, the intentional poisoning of America with a genetic weapon. I believe as do many others that this crime was committed on about 20% of those Americans injected. While this is a hypothesis, that a large number of our fellow citizens received placebo injections of saline (sterilized salt water), it seems pretty accurate likely. If you remember, only about one thousand six hundred Americans died in the first ninety days of the release of the mRNA shot by Pfizer in January of 2021. When you think about, had they injected all sixty-five percent of Americans with the real mRNA jab we would have seen a massive death and injury rate that would have crippled the entire country almost immediately causing the rest of the country to reject the jab without question. While somehow

Americans were OK about a million of them dying from this disease from 2021 to now, they wouldn't stand to keep taking the jab if the numbers were five times higher.

One of the things that always has bugged me about why FDA came at me so early in 2020. I present this explanation to you as the possible reason why: While all the other physicians who practiced early treatment of the Covid-19 infection beginning in the summer of 2020, I was already restoring health to almost everyone I treated from February of 2020, four months before a physician in an Emergency room in Southern California was able to do the same with hydroxychloroquine and zinc.

I see know that my actions were in some ways the biggest threat to Big Pharma while at the same time being the low lying fruit because I was a naturopathic physician practicing as a health coach. I had zero name recognition except to my existing patients, family and friends. I was certainly incapable financially of mounting a defense by bank-rolling a major law firm with a huge retainer. I sure learned first-hand how the federal courts, including the public defender's office are working with the same corrupt interpretation of the Constitution when and if they even refer to it at all. My attorneys it turned were like jesters at a royal castle. They were there to follow procedure to the letter, there to hold your hand when the case turned sideways on you and there to encourage you to do whatever the prosecutors, the judges, the jury and finally the Federal Bureau of Prisons decided. There defense NEVER had the strength of the constitution behind it because the judge didn't allow the jury to actually consider this contract we Americans have with the federal government.

Big changes need to occur in our country before justice and fairness can every return to the federal court system. We could be seeing that happen in this 2024 election cycle. On the other hand, it could turn out to be more of the same corruption by the same politicians we're so used to watching reduce our meager incomes with endless wars abroad they pay for by diluting the value of our dollars, weaken our health with more mRNA toxic jabs, and pollute us with aluminum and sulfur dioxide they spray into the high altitude skies in the name of Geo-engineering to "protect" us from global warming, without informing us or caring how it effects our health.

But even in these areas there is hope. The governor of Tennessee signed a bill in April, 2024 that forbids the spraying of these chemicals into their state skies. Eight other states are considering doing the same. A very large percentage of Americans, between 70-80% are refusing anymore mRNA jabs or boosters. It's getting better.

It's a historical fact that only three percent of the entire thirteen colonies every participated in the American Revolution. While the other ninety-seven percent may have heard that it was going on, both from a political and a military standpoint, it took only that very small amount of inspired, courageous and freedom loving colonists to win independence from King George and sovereignty for ALL Americans living in our country's early inception.

I welcome you to join the THREE PERCENTERS. Who knows what we can do with your help because today we have tools the colonists do not have. We live in the information age. We have smart phones, computers and we can hold on to our common sense and bring back the constitution of we want to.

Smiles! Rick Marschall ND

Health coaching somewhere on the Olympic Peninsula

Work Cited

1. Tips, Scott. "Never Has So Little Done So Much Harm to So Many." *Health Freedom News*, vol. 38, no. No. 1, 2020, p. 7.

2. Tips, Scott. "Never Has So Little Done So Much Harm to So Many." *Health Freedom News*, vol. 38, no. No. 1, 2020, p. 8.

3. Tips, Scott. "Never Has So Little Done So Much Harm to So Many." *Health Freedom News*, vol. 38, no. No. 1, 2020, p. 8.

4. Tips, Scott. "Never Has So Little Done So Much Harm to So Many." *Health Freedom News*, vol. 38, no. No. 1, 2020, p. 8.

5. https://www.nejm.org/doi/full/10.1056/nejme2002387

6. https://www.brown-watch.com/brownwatch-news/2021/8/4/sdsds

7. https://www.brown-watch.com/brownwatch-news/2021/8/4/sdsds

8. https://www.brown-watch.com/brownwatch-news/2021/8/4/sdsds

9. https://www.brown-watch.com/brownwatch-news/2021/8/4/sdsds

10. https://www.ncbi.nlm.nih.gov/pmc/articles/PMC9263052/#:~:text=Moreover%2C%20Nabil%20et%20al.',COVID%2D19%20%5B67%5D.

11. https://www.frontiersin.org/articles/10.3389/fmicb.2021.746795/full

12. https://www.ncbi.nlm.nih.gov/pmc/articles/PMC8274222/

13. https://www.webmd.com/lung/news/20210422/first-person-charged-under-covid-false-claims-law

14. https://journals.lww.com/americantherapeutics/fulltext/2021/08000/ivermectin_for_prevention_and_treatment_of.7.aspx

15. https://www.ncbi.nlm.nih.gov/pmc/articles/PMC8088823/

16. https://abc7.com/coronavirus-covid-19-chloroquine-hydroxychloroquine/6082485/

17. https://www.thedesertreview.com/opinion/columnists/open-letter-to-dr-anthony-fauci-regarding-the-use-of-hydroxychloroquine-for-treating-covid-19/article_31d37842-dd8f-11ea-80b5-bf80983bc072.html

18. https://www.medpagetoday.com/special-reports/exclusives/101529

19. https://childrenshealthdefense.org/
    https://www.amazon.com/Deluxe-Boxed-Set-Democracy-Childrens-ebook/dp/B09VQTK24G

20. https://www.google.com/search?q=judy+mikovits+books&rlz=1C1GCEA_enUS1041&oq=judy+mikovits+books&aqs=chrome..69i

57j0i22i30l4.6064j0j7&sourceid=chrome&ie=UTF-8

21. https://www.thriftbooks.com/w/ending-plague-a-scholars-obligation-in-an-age-of-corruption_kent-heckenlively_francis-w-ruscetti/26822381/item/55319164/?gclid=Cj0KCQiAlKmeBhCkARIsAHy7WVuL7ioh-MfThp10DGYl3PEJtYp4e2NRXD5I4o0_H-6gU_NF8TwC4e0aArYoEALw_wcB#idiq=55319164&edition=48673917

22. https://www.youtube.com/watch?v=k8RyV3VEDKI

23. https://rumble.com/v1wac7i-world-premier-died-suddenly.html

24. https://www.medrxiv.org/content/10.1101/2022.04.05.22273167v1.full

25. https://www.wnd.com/2021/06/fauci-funded-scientist-chinese-colleagues-created-killer-coronavirus/

26. https://www.congress.gov/117/meeting/house/114270/documents/HHRG-117-GO24-20211201-SD004.pdf

27. https://www.house.mi.gov/Document/?Path=2021_2022_session/committee/house/standing/workforce,_trades,_and_talent/meetings/2021-08-12-1/documents/testimony/Dr.%20Moehanid%20Talia.pdf   https://www.brown-watch.com/brownwatch-news/2021/8/4/sdsds

28. https://uploads-ssl.webflow.com/62f6c2ce87ee5b46474b4cf

5/62f75221d95bf7724d4a6132_The-Criminal-Conspiracy-of-Coronavirus.pdf

29. https://uploads-ssl.webflow.com/62f6c2ce87ee5b46474b4cf5/62f75221d95bf7724d4a6132_The-Criminal-Conspiracy-of-Coronavirus.p

30. https://www.wnd.com/2021/06/fauci-funded-scientist-chinese-colleagues-created-killer-coronavirus/

31. https://www.ncbi.nlm.nih.gov/books/NBK349040/

32. https://www.factcheck.org/2021/05/the-wuhan-lab-and-the-gain-of-function-disagreement/
https://www.newsweek.com/dr-fauci-backed-controversial-wuhan-lab-millions-

us-dollars-risky-coronavirus-research-1500741

33. https://uploads-ssl.webflow.com/62f6c2ce87ee5b46474b4cf5/62f75221d95bf7724d4a6132_The-Criminal-Conspiracy-of-Coronavirus.pdf

34. https://pubmed.ncbi.nlm.nih.gov/32756549/

35. https://rumble.com/vk4znu-2021-jul-09-fauci-pharma-rico-usa-manufactured-illusion.-dr-david-martin-wi.html

36. https://www.nationalreview.com/news/fauci-argued-benefits-of-gain-of-function-research-outweighed-pandemic-risk-in-2012-paper/

37. https://www.congress.gov/bill/117th-congress/senate-bill/3012/cosponsors?r=38&s=1
https://www.wsj.com/articles/covid-19-coronavirus-lab-leak-virology-origins-pandemic-11633462827

38. https://www.marshall.senate.gov/wp-content/uploads/ROM21985.pdf

39. https://www.forbes.com/sites/stevensalzberg/2022/10/24/gain-of-function-experiments-at-boston-university-create-a-deadly-new-covid-19-virus-who-thought-this-was-a-good-idea/?sh=73195d6a5ca3

40. https://childrenshealthdefense.org/defender/boston-university-scientists-engineering-viruses-labs-cola/

41. https://uploads-ssl.webflow.com/62f6c2ce87ee5b46474b4cf5/62f75221d95bf7724d4a6132_The-Criminal-Conspiracy-of-Coronavirus.pdf

42. https://www.youtube.com/watch?v=CSRnPgncs3Q

43. https://www.youtube.com/watch?v=CSRnPgncs3Q

44. https://www.thoughtco.com/forced-sterilization-in-united-states-721308#:~:text=1981,forced%20sterilization%20in%20U.S.%20history.

45. https://www.newyorker.com/books/page-turner/the-forgotten-lessons-of-the-american-eugenics-movement

46. Judy Mikovits et al, "End of Plague" (Children's Health Defense) page 256

47. https://link.springer.com/article/10.1007/s00392-022-02129-5

48. https://thetexan.news/dallas-cardiologist-peter-mcculloughs-medical-certifications-revoked-by-american-board-of-internal-medicine/

49. https://www.nwahomepage.com/news/patients-support-doctor-who-has-been-prescribing-ivermectin-to-inmates-with-covid-19/

50. https://www.medpagetoday.com/special-reports/exclusives/101529

51. https://www.organicconsumers.org/news/did-lockdowns-cause-increased-mortality-rates

52. https://www.ldnews.com/story/news/2022/02/03/lebanon-woman-touts-dr-edith-behr-to-prescribe-ivermectin-hydroxychloroquine/9313726002/

53. https://www.webmd.com/lung/news/20210422/first-person-charged-under-covid-false-claims-law

54. https://apnews.com/article/coronavirus-pandemic-health-business-worms-legislature-054e83c1a4d69704b4ed6508c301dd18

55. https://www.wesh.com/article/florida-doctor-claims-hes-treated-3000-covid-19-patients-with-human-version-of-ivermectin/39302154

56. https://www.medpagetoday.com/special-reports/exclusives/97237

57. https://www.imdb.com/title/tt1227378/?ref_=nm_knf_t_1

58. https://screencast-o-matic.com/player/c3X0DKVU47u

59. https://wmc.wa.gov/news/statement-charges-served-physician-license-ryan-cole

60. https://worldcouncilforhealth.org/multimedia/adverse-events-pregnancy-fertility/

61. https://phmpt.org/wp-content/uploads/2021/11/5.3.6-postmarketing-experience.pdf

62. https://www.pewtrusts.org/en/research-and-analysis/issue-briefs/2022/12/the-long-term-decline-in-fertility-and-what-it-means-for-state-budgets

63. https://live.childrenshealthdefense.org/chd-tv/shows/good-morning-chd/thankspfizer-the-mass-gaslighting-of-angelia-desselle/?utm_source=email&utm_medium=salsa&utm_campaign=CHD+TV&utm_term=chdtv&eType=EmailBlastContent&eId=5938c0e8-456c-4399-ae86-08b0a6f43f47

64. https://www.google.com/search?q=kirk+milhoan+md+covid&newwindow=1&rlz=1C1GCEA_enUS1043&sxsrf=AJOqlzXtUfPeAjrxXy3-6H_oibu6Glp-

gA%3A1675202308574&ei=BI_ZY9HSIv2H0PEP2OCDqAc&ved=0ahUKEwjR5J305vL8AhX9AzQIHVjwAHUQ4dUDCBA&uact=5&oq=kirk+milhoan+md+covid&gs_lcp=Cgxnd3Mtd2l6LXNlcnAQAzIFCCEQoAEyBQghEKABOgUIABCABDoGCAAQFhAeOgUIIRCrAjoICCEQFhAeEB1KBAhBGAFKBAhGGABQ6AJY5Q1glhFoAXAAeACAAV-IAawDkgEBNpgBAKABAcABAQ&sclient=gws-wiz-serp#ip=1

65. https://www.ncbi.nlm.nih.gov/pmc/articles/PMC8202656/

66. https://mail.google.com/mail/u/0/#inbox/FMfcgzGrcFhRtQclLwbWRrQmDGcCbGCL

67. https://www.dshs.texas.gov/covid-19-coronavirus-disease-2019/covid-19-vaccine-information

68. (https://youtu.be/v3cZ5wJ8Y9Q) https://www.youtube.com/watch?v=yVZ7hXt3Ya8
69. https://www.youtube.com/watch?v=1bfIoOiSrSQ

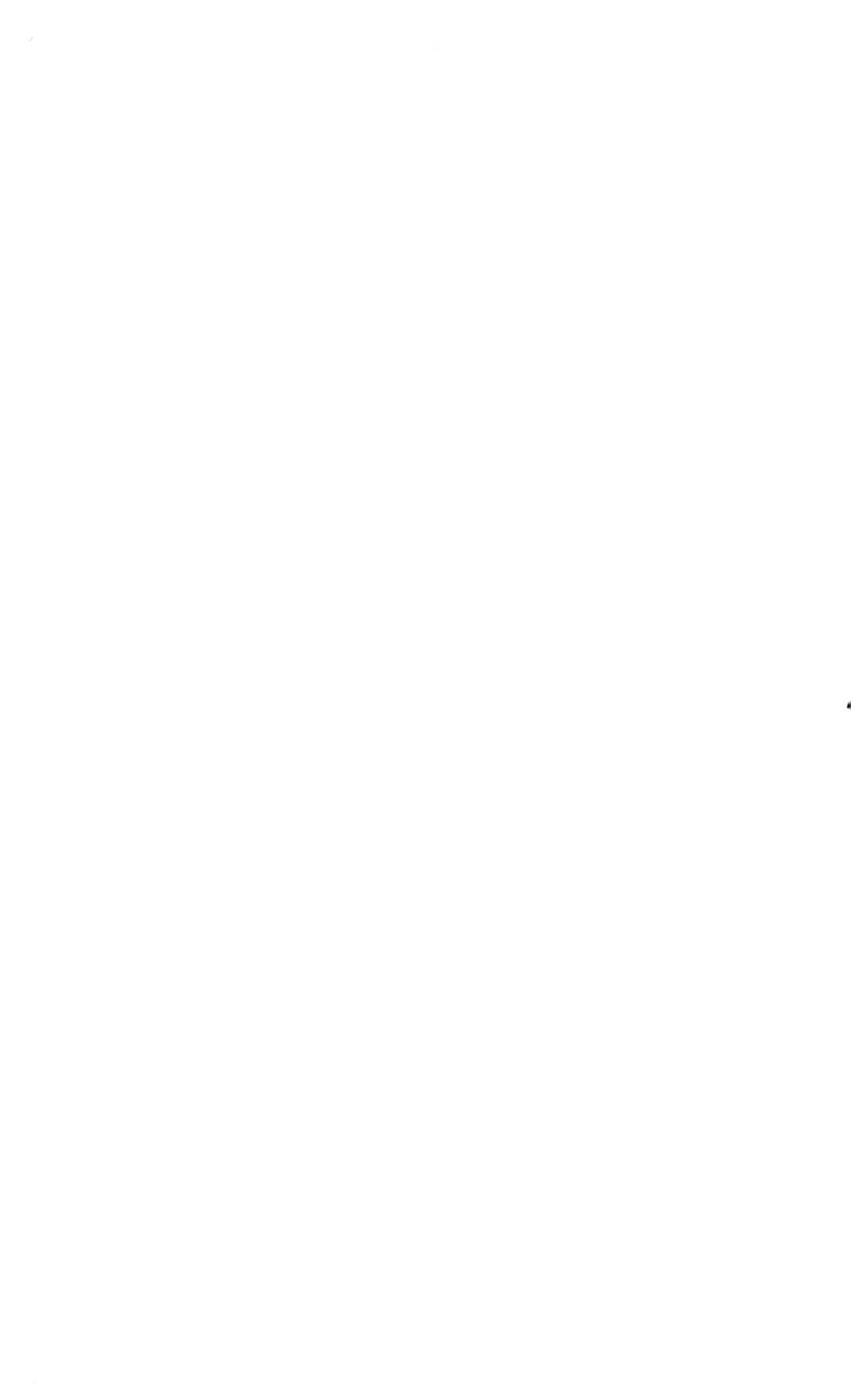

Made in United States
Troutdale, OR
10/07/2024